Evidence Synthesis
Number 109

Primary Care Screening for Abdominal Aortic Aneurysm: A Systematic Evidence Review for the U.S. Preventive Services Task Force

Prepared for:
Agency for Healthcare Research and Quality
U.S. Department of Health and Human Services
540 Gaither Road
Rockville, MD 20850
www.ahrq.gov

Contract No. HHS-290-2007-10057-I-EPC3, Task Order Number 3

Prepared by:
Kaiser Permanente Research Affiliates Evidence-based Practice Center
Kaiser Permanente Center for Health Research
3800 N. Interstate Avenue
 Portland, OR 97227

Investigators:
Janelle M. Guirguis-Blake, MD
Tracy L. Beil, MS
Xin Sun, PhD
Caitlyn A. Senger, MPH
Evelyn P. Whitlock, MD, MPH

AHRQ Publication No. 14-05202-EF-1
January 2014

This report is based on research conducted by the Kaiser Permanente Research Affiliates Evidence-based Practice Center (EPC) under contract to the Agency for Healthcare Research and Quality (AHRQ), Rockville, MD (Contract No. HHS-290-2007-10057-I-EPC3, Task Order Number 3). None of the investigators has any affiliations or financial involvement that conflicts with the material presented in this report. The findings and conclusions in this document are those of the authors, who are responsible for its contents, and do not necessarily represent the views of AHRQ. No statement in this report should be construed as an official position of AHRQ or of the U.S. Department of Health and Human Services.

The information in this report is intended to help health care decisionmakers—patients and clinicians, health system leaders, and policymakers, among others—make well-informed decisions and thereby improve the quality of health care services. This report is not intended to be a substitute for the application of clinical judgment.

This report may be used, in whole or in part, as the basis for development of clinical practice guidelines and other quality enhancement tools, or as a basis for reimbursement and coverage policies. AHRQ or U.S. Department of Health and Human Services endorsement of such derivative products may not be stated or implied.

This document is in the public domain and may be used and reprinted without permission except those copyrighted materials that are clearly noted in the document. Further reproduction of those copyrighted materials is prohibited without the specific permission of copyright holders.

Acknowledgments

The authors gratefully acknowledge the following individuals for their contributions to this project: Aileen Buckler, MD, MPH, and Tracy Wolff, MD, MPH, at AHRQ; Kirsten Bibbins-Domingo, MD, PhD, Mark Ebell, MD, MS, Jessica Herzstein, MD, MPH, and Albert Siu, MD, MPH, of the U.S. Preventive Services Task Force; Daphne Plaut, MLS, and Jonathan Fine, MFA, Maya Rowland, MPH, Brittany Burda, MPH, and Corinne Evans, MPP, at Kaiser Permanente Center for Health Research.

Suggested Citation

Guirguis-Blake JM, Beil TL, Sun X, Senger CA, Whitlock EP. Primary Care Screening for Abdominal Aortic Aneurysm: An Evidence Update for the U.S. Preventive Services Task Force. Evidence Synthesis No. 109. AHRQ Publication No. 14-05202-EF-1. Rockville, MD: Agency for Healthcare Research and Quality; 2014.

Structured Abstract

Objective: To assess the benefits and harms of AAA screening programs and approaches to treating small aneurysms, and to determine screening yield for subgroup populations.

Data Sources: We performed a search of MEDLINE, the Database of Abstracts of Reviews of Effects, and the Cochrane Collaboration Registry of Controlled Trials for studies published from January 2004 through June 1, 2012. We supplemented searches by examining bibliographies from retrieved articles, previous U.S. Preventive Services Task Force reviews, and consulting outside experts. We searched federal agency trial registries for ongoing and/or unpublished trials.

Study Selection: Two reviewers independently reviewed citations against a priori inclusion and exclusion criteria. Potentially relevant articles were then independently evaluated by two reviewers against the same inclusion criteria and quality-rated using U.S. Preventive Services Task Force criteria. Resolution of discrepancies occurred through discussion with a third reviewer. A single investigator extracted study characteristics and results into tables and a second reviewer checked accuracy.

Data Analysis: Evidence for all key questions (KQs) was qualitatively synthesized. Quantitative synthesis of outcomes for KQs 1, 3, 4, and 5 used a random-effects model as the primary analysis, with sensitivity analyses using a fixed-effects model. For KQ 1 only, additional sensitivity analyses were conducted using Peto odds ratios and hazard ratios, where reported.

Results: Based on four fair- to good-quality, population-based, randomized, controlled trials (RCTs) (N=137,214), one-time invitation for AAA screening in men age 65 years and older reduced AAA rupture and AAA-related mortality for up to 10 years, but had no effect on all-cause mortality after up to 15 years. Based on one fair-quality population-based RCT in women (N=9,342), screening had no AAA-related or all-cause mortality benefit. We found insufficient direct evidence to make conclusions about the yield of various high-risk screening approaches. We identified a group of heterogeneous, mostly small cohort studies examining rescreening yield that provided no clear data on which to base conclusions. Few studies addressed differences in rescreening yield by population subgroup or screening interval. Based on four fair-quality RCTs (N=137,214), invitation for screening was associated with some harms (i.e., more overall surgeries and more elective surgeries) but fewer emergency operations and decreased 30-day operative mortality at up to 10 to 15 years of followup. Four observational studies (N=1150) suggested no long-term quality of life difference from screening, although one study showed lower Short-form 36-item Health Survey scores at 6 weeks in the screened group, which did not persist.

Analysis of two good-quality RCTs (N=2,226) demonstrated that early open surgery compared with surveillance for small AAA (4 to 5 cm) decreased AAA rupture with attenuated benefit after 5 years, but did not alter AAA-related or all-cause mortality after up to 12 years of followup. One RCT showed no subgroup differences in all-cause mortality or AAA-related mortality by age, sex, or AAA diameter for open surgery versus surveillance. Open surgery compared with surveillance resulted in similar 30-day postoperative mortality and quality of life but fewer postoperative complications, particularly perioperative myocardial infarction. Meta-analysis of two underpowered fair-quality RCTs (N=1,088) of early EVAR compared with surveillance in small AAA found that EVAR does not reduce all-cause mortality, AAA-related mortality, or AAA rupture. EVAR complications reported in two RCTs and two registry studies (N=2,440) included systemic complications (15%), endoleaks (10%), and reintervention (4%) but no difference in operative mortality. One fair-quality RCT (N=339) suggested higher quality of life in early EVAR compared with surveillance in the first 6 months that did not persist at 3-year followup. A few fair-quality, small heterogeneous RCTs examined pharmacotherapy compared with surveillance for small AAA, with inconsistent results in altering AAA growth rates. There were few adverse reactions reported for antibiotics in these small trials but propranolol was poorly tolerated, leading to a high withdrawal rate.

Limitations: The four large population-based screening trials, while robust in numbers, almost exclusively represent a population of older Caucasian men from nonU.S. populations. Other than for age and sex, there is no direct evidence on AAA screening benefit for other subgroups by race, family history, smoking history, or cardiovascular risk. There is limited information on rescreening yield overall and by subgroup derived from one Department of Veterans Affairs trial. Two RCTs examining EVAR versus surveillance for small AAA were prematurely stopped due to futility analysis demonstrating less than 1 percent chance of finding a difference in AAA rupture or AAA-related mortality. These studies could be underpowered to detect other differences in health outcomes. The four RCTs addressing pharmacotherapy versus surveillance for AAA were small and studied heterogeneous populations. Quality of life studies examining possible harms from screening and treatment are small and examine outcomes at different time points in different populations.

Conclusions: One-time invitation for AAA screening in men ages 65 years and older was associated with decreased AAA rupture and AAA-related mortality but no difference in all-cause mortality. Treatment of small, screen-detected AAA with early open or EVAR surgery did not result in improved health outcomes compared with surveillance. Short-term but not long-term differences in quality of life have been seen with screening for AAA in those who screen positive.

Table of Contents

Figures

Tables

Appendixes

Chapter 1. Introduction

Scope and Purpose

The U.S. Preventive Services Task Force (USPSTF) commissioned this report to update the previous recommendation on abdominal aortic aneurysm (AAA) screening. In 2005, the USPSTF found good-quality evidence to recommend one-time screening for AAA by ultrasonography in men ages 65 to 75 years who have ever smoked (B recommendation).[1] The USPSTF concluded that the benefits of screening do not clearly outweigh the possible harms in men ages 65 to 75 years who have never smoked, and thus made no recommendation for or against screening for AAA in this population (C recommendation).[1] Also, based on the low prevalence of the condition and its sequealae and the presence of competing risks, the USPSTF recommended against routine screening for AAA in women age 65 years and older (D recommendation).[1]

This study applied systematic review methods to systematically assess the evidence regarding the benefits and harms of AAA screening and alternative strategies for managing screen-detected small AAA.

Background

Condition Definition

An AAA is a weakening in the wall of the abdominal section of the aorta, which is the largest artery in the body.[2] Once a section of the aortic wall is weakened, the pressure from the blood flowing through causes the aorta to bulge or balloon, resulting in the formation of an aneurysm.[3] A large proportion of AAAs are asymptomatic until the development of rupture. AAA rupture can be acute and is life-threatening.

The most accepted definition of an AAA is based on the diameter of the artery, with a diameter of 3.0 cm or larger considered to be an aneurysm.[4] This is more than two standard deviations (SDs) above the average diameter of the abdominal aorta (2.0 cm) in both men and women.[5] The abdominal aorta diameter varies somewhat by age, sex, and body size, which may influence the accuracy of this definition in some subgroups.[6] An AAA is also defined as a maximum infrarenal aortic diameter of at least 1.5 times larger than the expected infrarenal aortic diameter.[4] This definition, however, is less frequently used.

Prevalence and Burden of Disease

A number of population-based screening studies conducted in the United States, United Kingdom, Australia, Sweden, and Italy have shown that AAA affects 1.6 to 7.2 percent of the general population age 50 years and older.[7-16] Of note, in the past year, there have been several studies from established population-based screening programs in men age 65 years and older reporting declines in AAA prevalence in men over the past two decades in the United Kingdom,[17,18] New Zealand,[19] and Sweden,[11] with reported prevalence ranging from 1.5 to 1.7 percent. The prevalence differs substantially by sex (1.6% to 8.8% in men vs. 0.2% to 6.2% in women), and the ratio of prevalence is generally 4 to 15 times greater in men than women.[7,10,20] One recent study in 70-year-old women in Sweden reports a similar decline in the prevalence of AAA in women (approximately 0.4%).[11] The prevalence of AAA appears to increase with age. In the Western Australian study, for example, the prevalence is 4.8 percent in the population ages 65 to 69 years, 7.6 percent in ages 70 to 74 years, 9.7 percent in ages 75 to 78 years, and 10.8 percent in ages 80 to 83 years.[8] Ninety percent or more of identified aneurysms, however, are below the threshold for immediate surgery (3.0 to 5.5 cm).[8,9,11,21,22]

Each year, approximately 200,000 people are diagnosed with AAA in the United States, about 15,000 of whom develop AAAs large enough to be considered high risk for rupture.[3,23] A rupture is often fatal, and an estimated 59 to 83 percent of patients die prior to hospitalization.[24] The operative mortality (in-hospital or 30-day) of patients who survive until surgery has been estimated to be 41 percent. Thus, at most, 10 to 25 percent of individuals with ruptured AAAs survive to hospital discharge. Almost all deaths from ruptured AAAs occur after age 65 years.[25]

Data on the total societal economic burden of AAA are currently not available. Hospital discharge data show that patients with unruptured AAAs are hospitalized for an average of 6.7 days, presumably reflecting surgical treatment, with cumulative costs exceeding $59,000. In patients discharged after a ruptured AAA, the average hospital stay is 10.7 days and the average cost is more than $93,000.[26] The economic burden of AAA would be substantially larger if indirect costs (e.g., disability) were taken into account.

Etiology and Natural History

Although the direct causes for the development of AAA have not been fully understood, studies have suggested that smoking,[27,28] atherosclerosis,[29,30] and inflammation[31,32] may all contribute to the development of AAA. Genetic predisposition may also lead to AAA development, and polymorphisms in several genes associated with AAA development have been identified.[33,34]

While the expansion rate of AAAs can vary significantly, the reported average growth rate of aneurysms measuring between 3.0 and 5.5 cm is 0.2 to 0.3 cm annually.[4] The rate of expansion accelerates for larger aneurysms, ranging from a slow increase of 1.1 mm per year in ectatic aortas (2.5 to 2.9 cm in diameter)[35] to 4.9 mm per year for larger aneurysms (4.0 to 4.9 cm).[36] While a rapid rate of aneurysm expansion of more than 1 cm per year is commonly used in decisionmaking about elective repair of AAAs measuring smaller than 5.5 cm, the predictive value of expansion as an index of rupture risk is less clear.[37]

The annual risk of aneurysm rupture varies substantially. There is zero annual rupture risk for AAAs measuring between 3.0 and 3.9 cm, while aneurysms measuring 4.0 to 4.9 cm have a 1 percent annual rupture risk and those measuring 5.0 to 5.99 cm have an 11 percent annual rupture risk.[38-40] Although women have a much lower prevalence of AAA, they are two to four times more likely to have aneurysm rupture than men (based on the findings of a single study).[41]

Risk Factors

Risks Factors for Developing AAA

Significant risk factors for the development of AAA include advanced age,[42] male sex,[20] smoking,[4,43,44] and family history of AAA.[4,45,46] Other potential risk factors include a history of other vascular aneurysms,[47] taller height,[48] coronary artery disease,[48] cerebrovascular disease,[47] atherosclerosis,[48] hypercholesterolemia,[48] and hypertension.[4,48] In recent years, genomewide association studies have shown an association between AAA development and mutations on certain chromosomes, specifically chromosome 9p21.[4,49] Protective factors include African American race, female sex, and diabetes mellitus.[50]

Risk Factors for AAA Growth

A rigorous systematic review and individual patient data meta-analysis of 18 studies involving 15,475 patients examined the factors affecting the growth of small AAA.[51] Among all factors examined—including age, sex, smoking, body mass index, diabetes, arterial blood pressure, pulse pressure, and history of cardiovascular disease (CVD)—smoking was the only risk factor that was independently associated with the increased risk of small AAA growth (point growth rate, 0.35 [95% CI, 0.23 to 0.48 mm per year]), and diabetes was independently associated with lower risk of AAA growth (-0.51 [95% CI, -0.70 to -0.32 mm per year]). Age, sex, arterial blood pressure, pulse pressure, and history of CVD were statistically associated with AAA growth in unadjusted analyses; the apparent associations became nonstatistically significant in adjusted analyses.

Risk Factors for AAA Rupture

If the aneurysm is allowed to expand without intervention, or if the initial size of the aneurysm is large, the risk of aneurysm rupture is significant.[38,39,52-55] Older age, female sex, smoking, and higher arterial or pulse blood pressure are also associated with increased risk of rupture in patients with small AAA.[51] The rupture risk in women has been reported to be almost four times greater than the rupture risk in men (hazard ratio [HR], 3.76 [95% CI, 2.58 to 5.47]).[51] In addition, current smokers have been reported to have double the risk of aneurysm rupture than ever smokers or nonsmokers (HR, 2.02 [95% CI, 1.33 to 3.06]). Other potential pathogenic factors contributing to rupture include peak AAA wall stress[56,57] and a rapidly progressing expansion rate.[4,24,52,58]

Rationale for and Types of Screening/Screening Strategies

Identifying screening strategies that could reduce mortality and other adverse health outcomes is critical, since most AAAs are asymptomatic and have a high mortality rate if allowed to progress to rupture. Several strategies, including ultrasound, computed tomography (CT), and physical examination, may be used to identify AAA.

Ultrasonography is noninvasive, is easy to perform, and has high sensitivity (94% to 100%) and specificity (98% to 100%)[4,24,59-62] for detecting AAA. In addition, it has demonstrated high rates of reproducibility and is low in cost. In 1 to 3 percent of patients, however, it may be impossible to see the aorta due to bowel gas or obesity.[63,64] There are four aspects of aortic measurement: plane of acquisition, axis of measurement, position of calipers, and selected diameter. Trials vary in terms of reporting the specific technique, especially whether inner to inner wall versus outer to outer wall measurements are used.[65] Nevertheless, ultrasound screening has been widely accepted as the primary approach for detecting AAA by both primary care physicians and vascular surgeons.[4,24,44] The guidelines of both the Society for Vascular Surgery and the European Society for Vascular Surgery recommend ultrasound as the primary screening tool. Ultrasound has also been the primary modality studied in large population-based screening studies of AAA.[13,14,66,67]

CT scanning is another method that can be used to detect AAA. CT scans are more reproducible than ultrasound, but the size of the aneurysms detected by CT are generally 2 mm larger than that measured by ultrasound.[24,68] CT scans have also shown relatively high sensitivity (90%) and specificity (91%) for the detection of symptomatic AAA.[69] The Society for Vascular Surgery has recommended the use of CT scanning for operative planning due to its ability to determine the morphology of the AAA and the presence of renal arteries and occlusive disease.[24]

While physical examination for the detection of AAA has also been used in practice, such examinations have a low sensitivity. A good-quality case-control study estimated the sensitivity of detecting an AAA of 3.0 cm or larger to be 68 percent (95% CI, 60% to 76%), with a specificity of 75 percent (95% CI, 68% to 82%).[70] A meta-analysis of 15 cohort screening studies of asymptomatic patients estimated sensitivity to be even lower, at 39 percent.[71] This approach is not recommended for screening or preoperative planning.

Interventions/Treatment

The initial management options for a screen-detected AAA are defined by size. Patients with small AAAs (diameter of <5.5 cm) may receive regular surveillance or pharmacotherapy from their primary care physician, or are occasionally referred to vascular surgeons for elective surgery for rapid growth (e.g., 1 cm per year).[24] When the AAA diameter reaches 5.5 cm or larger, elective open surgery or endovascular repair (EVAR) is recommended.[4,24] Emergency surgery is needed for ruptured AAAs irrespective of diameter, although the risk of rupture of small AAA is very low.[38-40]

Interventions for Small AAA

A number of interventions exist for managing small AAA (i.e., 3.0 to 5.4 cm), including surveillance, pharmacotherapy, and, rarely, surgery (open or EVAR). Surveillance aims to monitor the expansion rate of the aneurysm and initiate surgery when the aneurysm reaches 5.5 cm.[4,24] Pharmacotherapy, a new treatment option for small AAA, is often used to slow aneurysm expansion. Currently used pharmaceutical agents include statins, angiotensin-converting enzyme (ACE) inhibitors, and antibiotics. Surgery, particularly EVAR, is an alternative treatment for small AAA.[72] The risk-benefit profile of EVAR, however, needs to be fully considered.

Interventions for Large AAA

Management strategies for large AAA (≥5.5 cm) include open surgery and EVAR to avoid rupture.[4,24,44] Open surgical repair, the conventional method for repairing large AAA, has been substantially tested in randomized trials.[24] Both the American and European Vascular Societies recommend open repair for aneurysms measuring larger than 5.5 cm.[4,24,44] In an open repair, a vascular surgeon opens a patient's abdomen and replaces the weakened section of the aorta with an aortic graft.[3,24] The graft is a sturdy plastic tube that allows blood to easily pass through the artery and eliminates much of the risk of future AAA rupture.[3,24] Open repair requires hospitalization for 4 to 7 days, and recovery typically takes 6 weeks to 3 months.

EVAR is an alternative option to repair large AAA.[73] First introduced in 1991,[74] this technique has largely replaced open surgical repair over the last decade, especially for uncomplicated aneurysm repairs. In the United States, the annual number of EVAR procedures has increased six-fold since 2000.[24] Less invasive than open repair,[3,24,73] EVAR is performed by threading catheters through the blood vessels to replace the weakened section of the aorta with an endovascular stent graft. The length of hospitalization is usually 2 to 3 days, and the overall recovery is typically shorter than recovery from open repair.[3]

EVAR has advantages over open surgery, such as reduction in operative time, avoidance of general anesthesia, less trauma and postoperative pain, and reduced blood loss, from both intact and ruptured AAAs.[4,24,73] However, it has a higher reintervention rate than open repair because the graft is more likely to not seal properly, causing blood to begin to refill the aneurysm.[3,4] Typically, patients require followup visits with either ultrasound or CT imaging scans at 1, 6, and 12 months after EVAR, followed by annual visits for the rest of their lives.[3,73,75] If the patient experiences frequent problems after EVAR, conversion to open repair may be necessary.[4]

Three major trials (EVAR trial 1,[76-78] Open Versus Endovascular Repair trial,[79] and Dutch Randomized Endovascular Aneurysm Management trial[78,80,81]) comparing open and endovascular repairs for large AAA have suggested that EVAR has lower operative mortality than open surgery. There is no significant difference, however, in all-cause and aneurysm-related mortality between the two surgeries at a median followup of 6 years, and EVAR has higher risk of complications and reinterventions than open surgery. Another major trial (EVAR trial 2) comparing EVAR versus surveillance for large AAA unfit for open surgery also suggested that EVAR did not reduce all-cause and aneurysm-related mortality after a followup of 5 to 10 years.[82,83]

Current Clinical Practice

Ultrasound is the primary technology used to screen patients for AAA.[4,24] It is preferred to both physical examination and CT scans because it is inexpensive and noninvasive, can be easily implemented by both primary care and specialty clinics, and has optimal sensitivity and specificity.[4]

Once an AAA is detected, the management of the aneurysm depends on its size, the risk of rupture, and the risk of operative mortality.[4] The current standard of care is to maintain ultrasound surveillance at regular intervals for patients with small AAAs (3.0 to 5.4 cm) because the risk of rupture is negligible.[4] The Society for Vascular Surgery recommends followup surveillance with ultrasound every 3 years for healthy patients with AAAs measuring between 3.0 and 3.4 cm in diameter, at 12-month intervals for AAAs measuring 3.5 to 4.4 cm in diameter, and at 6-month intervals for AAAs measuring between 4.5 and 5.4 cm in diameter.[24] According to the Society for Vascular Surgery, however, the quality of evidence supporting this recommendation is low.[24]

The universal standard for elective repair is that patients with AAAs with a diameter of 5.5 cm or larger should be referred to a vascular surgeon for surgical intervention with either open repair or EVAR.[4,24,44,73] This recommendation is based on randomized, controlled trials (RCTs) with populations consisting mainly of men; as a result, the aneurysm size needed for surgical intervention may be different in women.[4,73]

Previous USPSTF Recommendation

In 2005, the USPSTF found good evidence to recommend one-time screening for AAA by ultrasonography in men ages 65 to 75 years who have ever smoked (B recommendation). The USPSTF concluded that the benefits of screening did not clearly outweigh the harms in men ages 65 to 75 years who have never smoked and did not make a recommendation for or against screening for AAA in this population (C recommendation). The USPSTF recommended against routine screening for AAA in women (D recommendation).[1]

Previous USPSTF Conclusions

The USPSTF found good-quality evidence that screening for AAA and surgical repair of large AAA ($\geq$5.5 cm) in men ages 65 to 75 years who have ever smoked leads to decreased AAA-specific mortality. There was good evidence that ultrasound is an accurate screening test for AAA when performed in a setting with adequate quality assurance. There was also good-quality evidence of important harms of screening and early treatment, including an increased number of surgeries, with clinically significant morbidity and mortality, as well as short-term psychological harms. Based on the moderate magnitude of net benefit, the USPSTF concluded that the benefits of screening for AAA in men ages 65 to 75 years who have ever smoked outweighed the harms.[1]

The USPSTF also found good-quality evidence that screening for AAA in men ages 65 to 75 years who have never smoked leads to decreased AAA-specific mortality. There is, however, a lower prevalence of large AAA in men who have never smoked compared with men who have ever smoked; therefore, the potential benefit from screening in men who have never smoked is small. There was good-quality evidence that screening and early treatment led to important harms, including an increased number of surgeries, with associated clinically significant morbidity and mortality, and short-term psychological harms.

Based on the available evidence at the time of the recommendation statement, the prevalence of large AAA in women was determined to be low, leaving only a small number of AAA-related deaths that could be prevented by screening. There was good-quality evidence that screening and early treatment resulted in important harms, including an increased number of surgeries, with associated morbidity and mortality, and psychological harms. The USPSTF concluded that the harms of screening women for AAA outweighed the benefits.[1]

Chapter 2. Methods

Scope and Purpose

This systematic review will provide updated evidence regarding the effectiveness of one-time and repeated screening for AAA, the associated harms of screening, and the benefits and harms of available treatments for small AAA (3.0 to 5.0 cm) identified through screening. The USPSTF will use this review to update its 2005 recommendation for primary care practices. This review included all trials from the previous review that met current inclusion/exclusion criteria, as well as newly identified studies.[84]

Key Questions and Analytic Framework

Using the USPSTF's methods (detailed in **Appendix A**),[85] we developed an analytic framework (**Figure 1**) and five key questions (KQs).

The KQs include:

1. What is the effect of one-time AAA screening on health outcomes in an asymptomatic population age 50 years and older?
   a. Does the effect of one-time screening vary between men and women, smokers and nonsmokers, older (≥65 years) and younger (<65 years) patients, patients with and without a family history of AAA, and patients of different races/ethnicities?
   b. Does the effect of one-time screening vary between different screening approaches?
2. What is the effect of rescreening for AAA on health outcomes or AAA incidence in a previously screened, asymptomatic population without AAA?
   a. Does the effect of rescreening vary between men and women, sizes of AAA, smokers and nonsmokers, older (≥65 years) and younger (<65 years) patients, patients with and without a family history of AAA, and patients of different races/ethnicities?
   b. Does the effect of rescreening vary between different time intervals?
3. What are the harms associated with one-time and repeated AAA screening?
4. What is the effect of pharmacotherapy versus placebo or surgery (open and EVAR) versus surveillance on treatment-relevant intermediate health outcomes in an asymptomatic population with small AAA (3.0 to 5.4 cm) identified by screening?
   a. Does the effect of pharmacotherapy, surgery, and surveillance differ between men and women, smaller (3.0 to 4.0 cm) and larger aneurysms (4.1 to 5.4 cm), smokers and nonsmokers, older (≥65 years) and younger patients (<65 years), patients with and without a family history of AAA, patients with and without diabetes, patients with and without chronic obstructive pulmonary disease (COPD), or patients of different races/ethnicities?
5. What harms are associated with pharmacotherapy, EVAR and open surgery, and surveillance in an asymptomatic population with small AAA (3.0 to 5.4 cm) identified by screening?

Data Sources and Searches

In addition to considering all studies from the previous review for inclusion in the current review, we performed a comprehensive search of MEDLINE, the Database of Abstracts of Reviews of Effects, and the Cochrane Collaboration Registry of Controlled Trials for studies published between January 2004 and June 1, 2012. A bridge search was conducted through January 2013. We worked with a medical librarian to develop our search strategy (**Appendix B**). All searches were limited to articles published in the English language. The literature search results were managed using version 12.0 of Reference Manager® (Thomason Reuters, New York, NY).

To ensure the comprehensiveness of our retrieval strategy, we reviewed the reference lists of included studies and relevant systematic reviews and meta-analyses to identify relevant articles that were published before the timeframe of or not identified in our literature searches. In addition, we obtained references from outside experts. We also searched federal agency trial registries for ongoing and/or unpublished trials (**Appendix C**). We also used news and table-of-contents alerts from Google (Google, Inc., Mountain View, CA), and ScienceDirect (Elsevier, Maryland Heights, MO) to help us identify potentially eligible trials that were published between bridge searches.

Study Selection

Two reviewers independently reviewed the title and abstracts of all identified articles to determine if the study met the inclusion and exclusion criteria for design, population, intervention, and outcomes (**Appendix A**). Two reviewers then independently evaluated the full-text article(s) of all potentially included studies against the complete inclusion and exclusion criteria. Disagreements in the abstract and/or full-text review were resolved by discussion and consultation with a third reviewer if necessary. Excluded studies and reasons for exclusion are listed in **Appendix D**.

We developed an a priori set of criteria for inclusion and exclusion of studies based on our understanding of the literature (**Appendix A Table 1**). For KQs 1 and 2, examining the effectiveness of one-time and repeated screening, we considered RCTs and large cohort studies (n ≥1,000) of asymptomatic adult populations. For KQ 4, examining the effectiveness of treating small AAA, we considered only RCTs of asymptomatic adult populations with AAAs identified as small (3.0 to 5.4 cm). For KQs 3 and 5, examining the harms of screening for AAA and of treating small AAA, we were more inclusive and considered RCTs, observational and case-control studies, and registry data related to surgical harms. For KQ 5, we considered only populations of adults with asymptomatic small aneurysms. For all KQs, the only screening modality that we considered was ultrasound. We did not consider physical examinations due to literature reporting unfavorable sensitivity and specificity of this diagnostic method.[70] Further, we did not consider CT or magnetic resonance imaging screening, as these modalities are not readily available in primary care. For KQ 2, we accepted targeted screening defined as screening based on one or more patient risk factors or screening based on prediction/prognostic modeling. For KQs related to the treatment of small AAA, we considered surgical (open or EVAR) or pharmacotherapy interventions (statins, ACE inhibitors, beta-blockers, or antibiotics) compared with surveillance, usual care, or placebo. We limited included studies to those that were deemed good- or fair-quality by the USPSTF quality rating standards[86] and those published in English. Studies of poor quality and those not published in English were excluded. The outcomes that were reviewed are fully listed in **Appendix A Table 1**.

Quality Assessment of Evidence

Two reviewers independently assessed the methodological quality of each study using predefined criteria developed by the USPSTF[86] and supplemented with the National Institute for Health and Clinical Excellence methodology checklists for observational studies.[87] Disagreements in quality were resolved by discussion. Each study was given a final quality rating of good, fair, or poor.

Good-quality RCTs had adequate randomization procedures and allocation concealment, blinded outcome assessment, reliable outcome measures, similar groups at baseline (i.e., little to no statistically significant differences between groups in baseline demographics and characteristics), low attrition (≥90% of participants had followup data, with <10 percentage-point difference in loss to followup between groups), and used conservative data substitution methods if missing data were inferred. Trials were downgraded to fair if they were unable to meet the majority of the good-quality criteria. Trials were rated as poor quality if attrition was greater than 40 percent or differed between groups by 20 percentage points, or if there were any other "fatal" flaws that seriously affected internal validity, as agreed upon by two independent investigators. Poor-quality studies were excluded from the review (**Appendix D**).

Good-quality observational studies had an unbiased selection of the nonexposed cohort and adequate ascertainment of exposure. These studies addressed a population without the outcome of interest at the beginning of the study, and they had reliable outcome measures, blinded assessment, low attrition, adjustment for potential confounders, and no other important threats to internal validity. Observational studies were downgraded to fair if they were unable to meet the majority of good-quality criteria. Poor-quality observational studies had multiple threats to internal validity and were excluded from the review.

Data Extraction

One reviewer extracted data from all included studies rated as fair- or good-quality into a standard evidence table and a second reviewer checked the data for accuracy. Elements abstracted included population characteristics (e.g., baseline demographics, body mass index, concurrent conditions, family history of AAA, smoking status, and CVD risk factors), study design (e.g., recruitment procedures, inclusion/exclusion criteria, followup, and population adherence), intervention characteristics, and postscreening management, as well as health outcomes.

Health outcomes included the number of participants experiencing an event and incidence rates.

For KQs 1, 2, and 3 (efficacy and harms of screening), we abstracted the reported incidence and prevalence of AAA, incidence of ruptured aneurysms, and mortality (all-cause, AAA-related, and operative). In addition, we extracted information on the number and circumstance (i.e., emergency or elective) of surgical interventions reported in each study and any adverse events related to screening (e.g., changes in quality of life, anxiety) that were reported. For KQs 4 and 5 (efficacy and harms related to treating small AAA), we abstracted data related to the dose and duration of the pharmaceutical intervention, surgical details (if reported), AAA growth rate, the number and circumstance (i.e., emergency or elective) of surgical interventions, incidence of aneurysm rupture, and mortality (all-cause, AAA-related, and operative). For adverse events, we extracted all that were reported, but specifically looked for incidence of reinterventions, endoleaks, device migration, conversion to open surgery, and readmission to the hospital within 30 days of surgery.

Data Synthesis and Analysis

We synthesized data separately for each KQ. Specifically, we qualitatively summarized each of the included studies regarding study design and setting, internal validity and major factors threatening the internal validity, and important characteristics about patients and interventions.

Data Synthesis for KQ 1 (Benefits of Screening for AAA)

We examined all-cause mortality, AAA-related mortality, rupture, and emergent repairs for ruptures for the comparison of screening versus no screening. We used the DerSimonian and Laird random effects model as the primary analysis to pool trials.[88] All statistical testing was two-sided and 0.05 was considered significant. We analyzed risk ratios for all outcomes. We examined statistical heterogeneity across trials with the I^2 statistic and chi-square test of heterogeneity.

We undertook the following sensitivity analyses to check the robustness of results:

- We conducted fixed-effects meta-analyses for trials, and we qualitatively compared the results between the fixed- and random-effects model.
- We conducted random-effects meta-analyses of trials reporting HRs for all-cause mortality, AAA-related mortality, and rupture, and we qualitatively compared the pooled estimates using HRs versus risk ratios.
- We conducted meta-analyses of trials reporting AAA-related mortality using the Peto odds ratio (OR) method to address rare events and to see if there were any important changes in significance compared with the DerSimonian and Laird models.
- We examined long-term followup for all-cause mortality, AAA-related mortality, and AAA rupture using the outcome data reported at the latest followup.

We also applied funnel plots to examine publication bias for the main health outcomes, including all-cause mortality, AAA-related mortality, and AAA rupture.

Data Synthesis for KQ 2 (Benefits of Rescreening for AAA)

Because of substantial differences in patient population, length of followup, and outcomes reported, we were unable to pool studies. We thus qualitatively summarized data and reported outcomes, including incidence of AAA, AAA ruptures, AAA-related mortality, and all-cause mortality.

Data Synthesis for KQ 3 (Harms of One-Time Screening and Rescreening for AAA)

For the comparison of screening versus no screening, we examined 30-day mortality, 30-day mortality after elective surgery, 30-day mortality after emergency surgery, and overall number of operations, elective operations, and emergency operations. We used the DerSimonian and Laird random-effects model as the primary analysis to pool trials.[88] All statistical testing was two-sided and 0.05 was considered significant. We analyzed risk ratios for all outcomes. We examined heterogeneity across trials with the I^2 statistic and chi-square test of heterogeneity. To examine the robustness of pooled results, we also conducted fixed-effects meta-analyses for trials, and compared the results between the fixed- and random-effects model.

Because of the substantial difference in quality of life measurements and insufficient reporting of data (e.g., lack of variation parameters), we were unable to pool these data in the studies of screening versus no screening.

For the rescreening studies, we also qualitatively summarized 30-day mortality, number of AAA operations, and quality of life due to limited data and differences in patient population and length of followup.

Data Synthesis for KQs 4 and 5 (Benefits and Harms of Treatment of Small AAA)

We conducted meta-analyses of trials of open surgery versus surveillance and EVAR versus surveillance in the management of small AAA (3.0 to 5.5 cm).

Main Analyses

We conducted DerSimonian and Laird random-effects meta-analyses of trials reporting all-cause mortality, AAA-related mortality, AAA rupture, 30-day operative mortality, and surgical procedure use using the estimate of heterogeneity from the Mantel-Haenszel model. We had planned to use HRs as the measure of effect for pooling of trials for time to all-cause mortality, AAA-related mortality, and rupture, since the length of patient followup varied significantly within studies (e.g., 3 to 6 years in the U.K. Small Aneurysm Trial [UKSAT]) and because HR is the most appropriate measure of effect for time-to-event data. However, the time-to-event data were only available for pooling all-cause mortality. We thus reported pooled risk ratios for all outcomes, in addition to the pooled HR for all-cause mortality. For trials with zero events, we used a continuity correction of 0.5. All statistical testing was two-sided and 0.05 was considered significant. We examined heterogeneity across trials with the I^2 statistic and chi-square test of heterogeneity.

Exploration of Heterogeneity

Among all the prespecified hypotheses, data were available for exploring heterogeneity of effect only for all-cause mortality by AAA diameter at baseline and sex in two trials comparing open surgery versus surveillance. To undertake our subgroup analyses, we initially pooled the results of each subgroup across studies (e.g. data for males from both the UKSAT and the Aneurysm Detection and Management [ADAM] trial) and subsequently tested for the interaction across the subgroups.

Sensitivity Analyses

We undertook the following sensitivity analyses to check the robustness of results:

- For all-cause mortality, we conducted random-effects meta-analyses of trials reporting risk ratios, and we qualitatively compared the pooled estimates using HRs versus risk ratios.
- For those outcomes with a very low event rate (e.g., AAA-related mortality), we conducted fixed-effects meta-analyses, and we qualitatively compared the results between a fixed- and random-effects model.
- For trials with zero events, we used an alternative continuity correction (i.e., 0.005).

Because of the very small number of trials included in each of the meta-analyses, we did not apply funnel plots to examine the publication bias.

Additional Analyses

The data reported on adverse effects of open surgery and EVAR, such as quality of life and surgical complications, did not allow for quantitative analyses. We thus summarized these data qualitatively by the type of intervention (open surgery vs. EVAR) and adverse outcome.

USPSTF Involvement

This research was funded by the Agency for Healthcare Research and Quality (AHRQ) under a contract to support the work of the USPSTF. The authors worked with three USPSTF liaisons at key points throughout the review process to develop and refine the scope, analytic framework, and KQs; to resolve issues around the review process; and to finalize the evidence synthesis. AHRQ had no role in study selection, quality assessment, or synthesis. AHRQ staff provided project oversight, reviewed the draft evidence synthesis, and distributed the initial evidence report for external review of content by outside experts, including representatives of professional societies and federal agencies. The final published systematic evidence review was revised based on comments from these external reviewers.

Chapter 3. Results

Literature Search

Our literature search yielded 2,723 unique citations. From these, we provisionally accepted 204 articles for review based on titles and abstracts (**Appendix B**). After screening the full-text articles, 51 studies (68 articles) were judged to have met the inclusion criteria (**Appendix A**). The remaining 151 full-text articles were excluded (**Appendix D**).

Overview of Included Studies

Twenty-four studies, including 13 RCTs, eight cohort studies, and three case-control studies that were reported in 44 published papers, were included in our systematic review.[13-16,25,41,67,89-124] Of those studies, four major RCTs—two good- and two fair-quality—investigated the benefits of one-time screening for AAA in general asymptomatic populations;[13-16] these four studies and two additional fair-quality cohort studies also assessed harms associated with one-time screening for AAA.[104,105] No RCTs were available for assessing the effect of rescreening, but seven observational studies (six cohort studies and one case-control study) examined the benefits of rescreening,[96-102] and one of these also reported harms.[99] Additionally, two large, good-quality RCTs reported benefits and harms of early open surgery for small AAA,[106,108] and two moderate-sized, fair-quality RCTs assessed the benefits of early EVAR for small AAA.[113,115] Those two RCTs and two additional fair-quality registry studies also reported harms associated with early EVAR for small AAA.[122,123] Four small- to moderate-sized RCTs investigated the benefits and harms of beta-blockers and antibiotics for small asymptomatic AAA,[116,118-120] and one additional RCT reported harms associated with the use of beta-blockers.[117] Because of the complexity of the evidence body, we report information regarding study design, patient and intervention characteristics, and study outcomes about screening for AAA and treatment of small AAA, respectively.

KQ 1. What Is the Effect of One-Time AAA Screening on Health Outcomes in an Asymptomatic Population Age 50 Years and Older?

Summary of Results

Four large population-based screening RCTs of men age 65 years and older examined the effectiveness of one-time AAA screening, showing that AAA prevalence varies from 4 to 7.7 percent and the majority of screen-detected AAAs are small, measuring smaller than 4 to 4.5 cm. Invitation for screening in men age 65 years and older was associated with reduced AAA-related mortality, AAA rupture rates, and number of emergent surgeries but not all-cause mortality.

Study Details

Two fair-quality and two good-quality population-based screening RCTs from the United Kingdom, Denmark, and Australia assessed the efficacy of AAA screening in population-based settings: the Multicentre Aneurysm Screening Study (MASS) (n=67,800);[13,89,90,129] the Chichester, United Kingdom screening trial (n=15,775);[14,25,91,124] the Viborg County, Denmark screening trial (n=12,639);[15,67,92,93,125] and the Western Australian screening trial (n=41,000) (**Appendix E Table 1**).[16] All trials identified potential participants age 64 or 65 years and older from population registries or regional health directories. MASS identified participants from four centers in the United Kingdom, the Chichester trial included nine general practices in Chichester, the Viborg trial included the population from Viborg County, and the Western Australian trial included participants from a capital city and satellite towns. Reported mean (or median) ages ranged from 67.7 to 72.6 years, and the oldest study participants were age 80 years. One study, the Chichester trial,[14] included women,[25] while the other three recruited only men. Other than age and sex, no studies reported outcomes by any other demographic information. The Viborg trial reported AAA-related comorbidity risk factor information from hospital discharge data, indicating that 26.5% of all participants had at least one cardiovascular risk factor or COPD.[93,125] The Western Australian trial reported cardiovascular comorbidity and risk factor information for the screened group and analyzed the association between the risk factor and AAA diagnosis, but these risk factors were not collected for the control group, nor were they linked to mortality outcomes.[8] Three studies had no trial exclusions; only MASS excluded patients who 1) were identified by their primary care physician as too high risk to be screened, 2) were terminally ill, or 3) had other serious health problems or prior AAA repair.

All trials randomized participants to two groups: the control group received usual care, while the invited group received a letter invitation for one-time ultrasound screening (**Appendix E Table 1**). All trials considered normal aortic diameter to be smaller than 3 cm and defined AAA as 3.0 cm or larger. Three of the RCTs (MASS, Viborg, Chichester) further prescribed specific postscreening surveillance protocols for AAAs measuring 3.0 cm or larger with repeat ultrasounds,[13,14,67] while one trial (Western Australian) sent initial ultrasound results to primary care physicians for management.[16] In MASS, those with aortic diameters measuring 3.0 to 4.4 cm were rescanned yearly, those measuring 4.5 to 5.4 cm were rescanned at 3-month intervals, and those measuring 5.5 cm or larger were urgently referred to a vascular surgeon.[13] In the Viborg trial, individuals with ectatic aortic size of 2.5 to 2.9 cm were offered a repeat scan at 5 years, those measuring 3.0 to 4.9 cm were offered annual scans, and those measuring 5.0 cm or larger were referred to vascular surgery.[67] In the Chichester trial, patients with AAAs measuring 3.0 to 4.4 cm were rescanned annually, those measuring 4.5 to 5.9 cm were rescanned every 3 months, and those measuring 6 cm or larger were referred to a vascular surgeon, as were those with an increase in diameter of 1 cm or more per year.[14]

The primary outcome reported in trials was AAA-specific mortality (defined as all AAA deaths plus all deaths within 30 days of AAA surgical repair); all four trials also reported AAA rupture rate and all-cause mortality as benefit outcomes (**Appendix E Table 1**). Mortality data and causes of death were ascertained from death certificates in all studies, and three of the RCTs additionally involved an independent blinded review of autopsy reports and/or hospital records for all AAA-related deaths. Mean followup in these trials ranged from 3.6 to 15 years. Local and national health departments, research councils, and heart foundations funded these studies. MASS[13] and the Viborg trial[67] were assigned a good-quality rating based on USPSTF criteria.[86] MASS had the greatest number of participants and the highest adherence to screening, with clear reporting of randomization, allocation, blinding of outcome assessors, and confirmation of equal followup in the invited and control groups.[13] The Viborg trial, while the smallest, adequately reported randomization and blinding of outcome assessors. There was, however, a difference between attendees and nonattendees, with nonattendees being significantly older than attendees (one third of those age 73 years vs. <20% of those ages 65 to 67 years did not attend).[67] The Chichester and Western Australian trials were assigned fair-quality ratings due to inadequate description of blinding of outcome assessors and lack of reporting of loss to followup (Chichester) or lack of detail regarding randomization method (Western Australian).[14,16] All trials appeared to use intention-to-treat analysis; adherence to screening varied from the lowest adherence in the Western Australian trial (62.5% of those invited attended screening) to the highest adherence in MASS (80.2% adherence). All studies reported outcomes for attendees and nonattendees in the invited group separately. Three studies reported low loss-to-followup rates in the participants with AAA: MASS (72% at 10-year followup),[13] Viborg trial (75.1% retention rate in invited group; 58.0% in control group at 52-month followup),[67] and Western Australian trial (87.1% retention in invited group; 84.9% in the control group at 3.6-year followup).[16]

AAA Prevalence in the Screened Population

AAA prevalence on the initial screening for male attendees varied from 4.0 and 4.9 percent in the Viborg trial and MASS to 7.6 and 7.7 percent in the Chichester and Western Australian trials, respectively (**Table 1**). The two latter trials with higher AAA prevalence rates recruited older participants (Chichester median age, 72 years; Western Australian mean age, 72.7 years; compared with mean ages of 67.7 and 69.2 years in the Viborg trial and MASS, respectively). Three of the four trials (MASS, Chichester, and Western Australian) reported prevalence of AAA by size at initial screening. MASS and the Western Australian trial reported that the majority of AAAs (71% to 80%) were small, measuring 3.0 to 4.4 cm. In Chichester, approximately 60 percent of the detected AAAs were 3.0 to 3.9 cm. The prevalence of larger AAAs (≥5 cm or ≥5.5 cm) in the screened population was consistent across studies and was reported as 0.4 to 0.6 percent (**Appendix F**).

Effect of Population Screening on AAA-Related Mortality

Table 2 presents the mortality results of the four population-based screening RCTs for men. MASS and the Viborg trial found statistically significant AAA-related mortality benefit in the invited group compared with the control group at each of the followup time points, while the Western Australian and Chichester studies had ORs/HRs of less than 1, but were not statistically significant. In these four trials, 26.3 to 77.4 percent of AAA-related deaths in the invited group occurred in nonattendees; however, all results used intention-to-treat analysis.

Meta-analysis of the four trials, using a random-effects model (**Figure 2**), produced a summary risk ratio (RR) of 0.57 (95% CI, 0.44 to 0.72), 0.38 (95% CI, 0.17 to 0.86), and 0.50 (95% CI, 0.31 to 0.79) in favor of screening at 3 to 5 years, 6 to 7 years, and 10 to 11 years, respectively. Pooled analysis of the three longest studies at 13 to 15 years (Chichester, MASS, and Viborg;

n=86,446) likewise showed a statistically significant benefit with AAA screening (RR, 0.58 [95% CI, 0.39 to 0.88]). High heterogeneity was detected at all time points after the 3- to 5-year time period, making the point estimate less reliable. Nonetheless, qualitative synthesis shows AAA-related mortality benefit appears as a consistent and persistent result over time when examining the individual trial results. Sensitivity analysis using HRs versus RRs and Peto ORs versus RRs did not alter conclusions (additional meta-analyses are shown in **Appendix K**). No publication bias was identified (**Appendix K**).

Effect of Population Screening on All-Cause Mortality

Each trial, except Viborg at 5.9 years, demonstrated no statistically significant benefit in all-cause mortality for men in the invited versus control group at each followup time point (**Table 2**).

Meta-analysis performed at four different time points ranging from 3 to 5 years up to 15 years of followup demonstrate no all-cause mortality benefit with an invitation for AAA screening compared with control (**Figure 3**). At the 15-year followup, pooled analysis from the longest trials, Chichester, MASS, and Viborg (n=86,446), produced a summary RR of 0.98 (95% CI, 0.97 to 1.00) using a random-effects model. Sensitivity analyses, performed using a fixed-effects model, changed the 6- to 7-year followup results to be statistically significant (OR, 0.96 [95% CI, 0.93 to 0.99]), and sensitivity analysis using studies with HRs as the measure of effect found a statistically significant reduction in overall mortality at 10 to 11 years (HR, 0.97 [95% CI, 0.95 to 0.99]) and at 13 to 15 years (HR, 0.97 [95% CI, 0.96 to 0.99]) (**Appendix K**). No publication bias was detected (**Appendix K**).

Effect of Population Screening on AAA Rupture

Individual study results for AAA rupture rate in men at different followup endpoints are presented in **Table 1** and **Figure 4**. Only MASS shows fewer AAA ruptures in the invited group at 4.1-year (RR, 0.51 [95% CI, 0.38 to 0.69]), 7-year (RR, 0.53 [95% CI, 0.43 to 0.65]), 10.1-year (RR, 0.52 [95% CI, 0.43 to 0.62]), and 13.1-year followup (RR, 0.57 [95% CI, 0.49 to 0.67]). At 4.3 years of followup, one of three trials (Viborg) showed a statistically significant reduction in AAA rupture. The Chichester trial showed fewer AAA ruptures at 5 and 10 years but not at 15 years. At 10 years, the Viborg and Chichester trials and MASS showed a benefit from screening. Using a random-effects model, meta-analysis demonstrated that screening was associated with a lower AAA rupture rate at all except the 15-year followup: 3 to 5 years (RR, 0.52 [95% CI, 0.35 to 0.79]), 7 years (RR, 0.53 [95% CI, 0.43 to 0.65]), and 10 to 11 years (RR, 0.27 [95% CI, 0.11 to 0.65]). Of note, despite MASS results included in the 13- to 15-year pooled analysis, there was still no statistically significant benefit in rupture at the 15-year followup. Heterogeneity was high at all time points; therefore, the magnitude of screening benefit on rupture is less certain. Sensitivity analyses using a fixed-effect model did alter the 13- to 15-year point estimate (RR, 0.61 [95% CI, 0.53 to 0.70]); sensitivity analysis using HRs did not alter conclusions (**Appendix K**). No apparent publication bias was found (**Appendix K**).

Emergent Repairs for AAA Rupture

Three trials reported rates of emergent AAA repairs for rupture in men in the invited and control groups (**Table 1**). Two of the three trials (Viborg and MASS) showed fewer emergency surgeries in the invited group at all measured time points. Meta-analysis using a random-effects model showed fewer emergent surgeries for AAA rupture at 3 to 5 years (RR, 0.42 [95% CI, 0.28 to 0.64]) (**Figure 5**). Pooled point estimates at the 13- to 15-year followup of the Viborg trial and MASS showed a reduction in emergent repairs in the invited group (RR, 0.42 [95% CI, 0.32 to 0.54]). Sensitivity analysis using fixed- versus random-effects models did not substantially alter results.

KQ 1a. Does the Effect of One-Time Screening Vary Between Men and Women, Smokers and Nonsmokers, Older and Younger Patients, Patients With and Without a Family History of AAA, and Patients of Different Races/Ethnicities?

Summary of Results

Only one population screening RCT examined AAA screening in women, showing that there is a low prevalence of AAA in women and that most AAAs detected at screening are small. There was no difference in AAA rupture rates at 5- and 10-year followup or in all-cause mortality at 5 years between the invited and control groups. Rupture rate is low, and most AAA ruptures occur in women age 80 years and older.[14,25]

Subanalyses from one RCT addressing ages younger and older than 65 years showed similar AAA-related or all-cause mortality benefit from screening in the older and younger screened age groups.[93] Another subanalysis from one RCT showed no AAA-related mortality benefit from screening in patients age 75 years and older or in those ages 65 to 74 years.[16]

Study Details

Women

Only the Chichester study recruited female participants ages 65 to 80 years (59% of participants were women; n=9,342 women) (**Appendix E Table 2**). Sex-specific results at 5-year followup are reported with the larger trial results;[14] 5- and 10-year sex-specific results are published separately.[25] Compared to men in every age cohort, more invited women refused screening. For example, in the 65-year-old cohort, 27.3 percent of invited women refused screening compared with 19.5 percent of men; in the 76- to 80-year-old cohort, 41.7 percent of invited women refused screening, while 33.8 percent of men refused. Prevalence of AAA in screened women was six times lower than that reported in Chichester men (1.3% vs. 7.6%, respectively) (**Table 1**). In the screened group, no women were diagnosed with AAA at the age of 65 years, 1 percent were diagnosed at ages 66 to 70 years, 1.8 percent at ages 71 to 75 years, and 1.6 percent at ages 76 to 80 years. The majority of AAAs (30/40) were small, measuring 3 to 3.9 cm; six AAAs measured 5.0 cm or larger. There was no difference in AAA rupture rates between the invited and control groups at 5- or 10-year followup (**Table 1**). At 5 years, three ruptures occurred in the invited group (0.06%) and three ruptures occurred in the control group (0.06%). At 10 years, 10 ruptures occurred in the invited group (0.21%) and nine ruptures occurred in the control group (0.19%). AAA-specific mortality was low in both groups (four deaths [0.08%] in the invited group and nine deaths [0.19%] in the control group; no statistical analysis) (**Table 2**). AAA-related mortality was reported in the entire unscreened population in Chichester, and while more than half of the AAA deaths in men occurred before age 80 years, the majority (70%) of AAA deaths in women occurred at age 80 years and older. All-cause mortality at 5 years was similar in both groups: 10.7 percent in the invited group and 10.2 percent in the control group. All-cause mortality was not reported for women at 10-year followup.

Older Adults

The oldest participants in the four major screening trials ranged in age from 73 to 80 years (**Appendix E Table 2**). Two of the population-based screening trials reported AAA-related mortality outcomes stratified by age or provided a subgroup analysis by age.[16,93] The 13-year followup of the Viborg trial performed a subgroup analysis of 5,429 men ages 64 to 65 years and showed similar AAA-related mortality benefit in the 64- to 65-year-old group (HR, 0.36 [95% CI, 0.14 to 0.93]) compared with the 66- to 73-year-old group (HR, 0.33 [95% CI, 0.18 to 0.62]).[93] Likewise, the lack of all-cause mortality benefit from screening was similar in the younger and older age groups (HR, 0.98 [95% CI, 0.89 to 1.07] in 64- to 65-year-olds; HR, 0.98 [95% CI, 0.93 to 1.03] in 64- to 73-year-olds). Of note, these subanalyses were not sufficiently powered. The Western Australian trial showed no AAA-related mortality benefit in the invited group age 75 years and older (OR, 1.13 [95% CI, 0.56 to 2.29]) or in those ages 65 to 74 years (OR, 0.82 [95% CI, 0.37 to 1.84]).[16]

None of the population-based screening RCTs reported smoking history, AAA family history, or race/ethnicity descriptive data for participants (**Appendix E Table 2**). All studies were conducted in majority Caucasian populations.

KQ1b. Does the Effect of One-Time Screening Vary Between Different Screening Approaches?

Summary of Results

One of the population-based RCTs collected risk factor information after randomization and analyzed AAA prevalence, AAA-related mortality, and overall mortality comparing low- and high-risk screening strategies. This simulation showed that there is a tradeoff: high-risk screening reduces the number of patients screened but prevents only half of AAA deaths.[93,125] This simulation used study methods that could lead to underascertainment of high-risk status, which would bias the estimated impact of high-risk screening toward a lesser effect.

Study Details

High-Risk Versus Low-Risk Screening Strategy

The Viborg trial collected risk factor information on all participants after trial randomization and analyzed the yield of high- and low-risk screening approaches based on comorbidity with 5- and 13-year followup in men ages 64 to 73 years.[93,125] The high-risk group included participants with one or more of the following conditions: hypertension, myocardial infarction (MI), COPD, ischemic heart disease, peripheral occlusive arterial disease, stroke, or transient ischemic attack. The low-risk group did not have any of the above comorbidities. The presence of comorbidities was extracted from hospital discharge diagnoses. Attendance in the high-risk group was significantly higher than in the low-risk group (78.8% vs. 75.8%, respectively; p<0.001).

Forty-six percent of the AAAs diagnosed in all participants (invited plus control) were in the high-risk group. In the screened group, prevalence of AAA in the high-risk group was more than double that of the low-risk group (6.7% vs. 2.9%). AAA-related mortality and total deaths were reported for each high-risk group, showing that the highest AAA-related mortality rate in the control group was in subgroups with peripheral artery disease (PAD) and COPD (AAA-related mortality, 4.62 vs. 3.42 per 1,000 years, respectively). Out of 339 patients with PAD, 157 died in the mean followup period of 5.1 years; one patient died of AAA-related causes in the invited group and four AAA deaths occurred in the control group. Out of 860 patients in the COPD group, 372 died at 5.2-year mean followup; one patient died of AAA-related causes in the invited group and seven AAA deaths occurred in the control group.

Kaplan Meier estimates over 8 years of followup showed that invitation for screening similarly reduced AAA-specific mortality in both low- and high-risk groups (HR, 0.24 [95% CI, 0.09 to 0.63] vs. 0.22 [95% CI, 0.08 to 0.65], respectively).

At 5-year followup, of the 30 AAA-related deaths that were prevented in the mass screening trial, selective high-risk screening would have prevented nearly half (14/30) of those deaths, and high-risk screening would have required 72.9 percent fewer screening invitations compared with mass screening. On the other hand, low-risk screening (only screening those without any of the risk factors) would have prevented about half (16/30) of the AAA deaths in the whole mass screening.

At 13-year followup, however, the high-risk AAA population realized less of an AAA-related mortality benefit from screening compared with the low-risk group (HR, 0.42 [95% CI, 0.2 to 0.87] vs. 0.29 [95% CI, 0.14 to 0.6], respectively). Results showing diminished benefit in the high-risk group at 13 years should be interpreted cautiously, as the Viborg trial's independent end point committee found classification bias, in which deaths of participants with known heart disease and AAA were more likely to be attributed to heart disease than to AAA. The effects of screening were therefore diminished, especially in the high-risk population with a high prevalence of coronary disease. At 13-year followup, there was no overall mortality benefit from invitation for screening (HR, 1.04 [95% CI, 0.95 to 1.13]).

Care should be taken in drawing definitive conclusions about high-risk screening yield based on this study. Because comorbidities were extracted from hospital discharge data, the high-risk cohort was likely sicker (i.e., required hospitalization) than a population defined as having one or more risk factors, thereby potentially biasing results against targeted, high-risk screening. For example, many participants in the Viborg trial with hypertension, PAD, or COPD would never have been hospitalized and therefore would never have been defined as high risk. Also, it is important to note that this was a simulation study; participants were randomized in the trial prior to risk factor collection or analysis, thereby making this study similar to a cohort study rather than an RCT.

There are no population-based screening trials comparing low- and high-risk screening approaches.

KQ 2. What Is the Effect of Rescreening for AAA on Health Outcomes or AAA Incidence in a Previously Screened, Asymptomatic Population Without AAA?

Summary of Results

Five fair-quality and one good-quality prospective cohort studies and one fair-quality case-control study with various rescreening protocols showed that AAA-related mortality over 5 to 12 years is rare (<3%) among those with normal aortas (<3 cm) on the initial scan.[96-102] Over 5 to 12 years, very few of those with aortas measuring smaller than 3 cm, particularly smaller than 2.5 cm, developed any AAA. As one would expect, some (19% to 88%) of those with initial diameters of 2.5 to 2.9 cm progressed to a diameter larger than 3.0 cm after 5 to 6 years. A smaller percentage grew to larger than 5 cm (0% to 2.4%) at 5 years,[98,100,126] and 15% had progressed at 10 years.[17] One fair-quality individual patient data meta-analysis reported data on time-to-event for AAA incidence and rupture for a subgroup of patients with subaneurysmal aortic dilatation (2.5 to 2.9 cm), also called ectatic aorta.[127] Mean time to rupture (after initial subaneurysmal detection) was 18.7 years (95% CI, 18.3 to 19.1) and was quite rare (<1%), although 8.3 percent developed a large aneurysm (≥5.4 cm) over a mean of 13.2 years.

A small number of participants with normal aortas were included in these studies, there are no matched controls in most studies, and most studies measured expansion rates rather than health outcomes.

Study Details

Five fair-quality and one good-quality prospective cohort studies[96-99,101,102] and one fair-quality case-control study[100] (two in the United States, four in the United Kingdom, and one in Denmark), with the number of total participants ranging from 223 to 15,098 and with mean followup ranging from 4 to 12 years, examined the yield of rescreening participants with normal or ectatic aortas (**Appendix G Table 1**).[96-103] Four of these trials recruited patients from subsets of larger population-based screening and treatment RCTs described in KQs 1 and 4.[96,99-101] The largest two studies were subsets of a screening RCT (n analyzed=4,308; subset from the

Chichester trial)[99] and a treatment trial (n analyzed=5,151; subset from the ADAM trial).[101] Definitions of normal and ectatic aortas differed; inclusion criteria based on aortic diameter were defined as follows: 2.5 to 2.9 cm,[96,100] 2.6 to 2.9 cm,[98] smaller than 2.6 cm,[102,103] smaller than 3 cm,[97,99] or 3 cm and larger.[101] Ultrasound measurement techniques varied, with some measurements obtained using inner-to-inner wall measurements,[17,99,126] outer-to-outer wall measurements,[96,100,101] or by unspecified measurements.[98] Repeat screening occurred at various intervals after the initial normal scan, as follows: 3 months to annually,[98] annually,[96] at 5 years and 12 years,[102,103] every 2 years for up to 10 years or once after 5 years,[99] once at 4 years,[101] once at 3 to 5 years,[100] and every 2 years.[97] While three of these trials also analyzed the yield of various surveillance strategies for small AAA (≥3 cm), these data are not reviewed here.[97,99,100] One individual patient data meta-analysis examined the subgroup with ectatic or subaneurysmal aortic diameters (2.5 to 2.9 cm) using time-to-event data for 1,696 individuals (66 women) from eight European centers.[127] Median age at first scan was 66 years (range, 56 to 71 years); period of followup varied (median, 4 years [range, 0.1 to 19.0]), as did mean number of scans per individual (2.0 to 6.7). Benefit outcomes reported in these trials included all-cause mortality,[17,96] AAA-related mortality,[17] AAA rupture (fatal and nonfatal),[17,96,97,101-103,126] and AAA growth rate.[98-100,102,103,126] Four of these studies reported use of procedures.[17,96,100,101]

Patient characteristics are shown in **Appendix G Table 2**. Studies included men age 65 years and older, with only one study including men as young as age 50 years.[101,127] Mean age was reported in four of the studies and ranged from 65.6 to 74.8 years,[96,98,99] with most studies averaging 65 to 68 years and one study with an older population mean age of 74.8 years.[98] Only one study reported inclusion of female participants (2.4%), and a few women (N=66) were included in the patient-level meta-analysis.[101] While one other study followed a subset of ADAM patients, there is no mention of the sex of participants; however, there cannot be a large number of women, given the low number of women in the original cohort.[96] Only the two studies which followed subgroups from the ADAM trial included risk factor information, including smoking history, family history, diabetes, COPD, hypertension, peripheral vascular disease, and CVD risk factors.[96,101]

AAA Incidence (New Cases)

Each study reported the percentage of participants with initially normal scans who eventually developed an AAA measuring 3.0 cm or larger during the 5- to 12-year followup period (**Table 3**). This AAA incidence varied considerably from 1 to 88 percent,[96-103] with the highest incidence of 88 percent found in the study with older participants (mean age, 74.8 years) who had an aortic measurement of 2.6 to 2.9 cm on their original scan.[98] Half or more of the incident AAAs were small, measuring 3 to 3.9 cm; in almost all studies, only 0 to 1.3 percent of normal AAAs (<2.5 or <3.0 cm) expanded to larger than 5 cm during the followup period. In a study of 547 men with an initial measurement of 2.6 to 2.9 cm, 15 percent developed an AAA larger than 5.4 cm over 10 years.[17] Based on individual patient data meta-analysis of 1,696 individuals (6 women) with subaneurysmal aortic diameters, 1,011 (59.6%) developed an AAA (≥3 cm) after a mean followup of 4.7 years (median followup, 4.0 years [range, 0.1 to 16.3 years]), while 8.3 percent developed a large AAA (>5.4 cm) after a mean followup of 13.2 years (median, 12.6 years [range, 1.2 to 19.5 years]).[127]

AAA Rupture

Reported AAA rupture rates were low in participants with ectatic or normal aortas (**Table 3**). Studies that included an initial diameter smaller than 2.6 or 3.0 cm reported no ruptures at 4 to 12 years.[101-103] A small study of 223 patients with an initial aortic diameter of 2.5 to 2.9 cm reported no AAA ruptures at 5.9-year mean followup,[96] but a study of 547 patients with initial aortic diameter of 2.6 to 2.9 cm reported that 2.4% had experienced a rupture at 10 years.[17] An individual patient data meta-analysis found AAA rupture to be rare (14/1,631).[127] A study of 2,691 men with an initial normal aorta reported a 0.07 percent rupture rate (95% CI, 0.02 to 0.30) at 10-year mean followup. The denominator for this rate included a population of patients who were screened once plus a population rescreened every 2 years for 10 years, so it is unclear whether these two ruptures occurred in the rescreened population.[97]

AAA-Related Mortality

AAA-related mortality rates ranged from 0 to 2.4 percent (**Table 4**). One study reported no AAA-related deaths at 5- and 12-year followup for those with an initial diameter of smaller than 2.6 cm.[102,103] Two studies followed a population of patients with an initial diameter of 2.6 to 2.9 cm and although there were no AAA-related deaths at 5 years, 2.4% had died of AAA-related causes at 10 years.

All-Cause Mortality

All-cause mortality was not well reported in these studies, but one study of individuals with an initial aortic diameter of 2.6 to 2.9 cm reported that 34% had died at 10 years.[17]

AAA Procedures

Several studies reported no AAA procedures at 4 to 5.9 years,[96,100,101] but one study of 547 participants with an initial aortic diameter of 2.6 to 2.9 cm reported that 11.5% had undergone a procedure by 10 years.[17] Most of these procedures were elective (9.7%).

Operative Mortality

Only one trial reported 30-day operative mortality (11.1%), and most deaths occurred in those with ruptured aortas (**Table 4**).[17]

KQ 2a. Does the Effect of Rescreening Vary Between Men and Women, Sizes of AAA, Smokers and Nonsmokers, Older and Younger Patients, Patients With and Without a Family History of AAA, and Patients of Different Races/Ethnicities?

Summary of Results

Only two prospective cohort studies (one fair-quality, one good-quality) analyzed AAA detection and AAA-related mortality rates with rescreening using uni- or multilogistic regression models by risk factor; both are subsets of the ADAM trial.[96,101] There were no AAA ruptures or AAA-related deaths in participants with normal aortas on initial screening in either of these studies. For detection rates with rescreening at 4 and 5.9 years, results are conflicting: one smaller cohort study (N=223) showed no association between risk factors and subsequent AAA detection, while the other, much larger, cohort (N=2,622) showed three risk factors (current smoker, coronary artery disease, and any atherosclerosis) associated with AAA detection at rescreening. One fair-quality cohort study examined the association between age of participants with aortic size smaller than 3.0 cm at initial scan and later development of AAA and found no association between age group and AAA-related mortality. Conclusions about the yield of rescreening in subgroups is limited by very few nonwhite or female participants and by the use of national death certificate information only for mortality data.

Study Details

A good-quality prospective cohort study involved a random subset of 5,151 veterans with normal aortas at initial screening who were offered rescreening at 4 years (subset of the ADAM trial) and given questionnaires about risk factor information.[101] Of those invited, 2,622 were rescreened. Participant information on 17 characteristics was collected: age, sex, race, height, weight, waist circumference, family history, smoking history, hypertension, hypercholesterolemia, coronary artery disease, claudication, cerebrovascular disease, deep venous thrombosis, diabetes, COPD, and nonskin cancer. This cohort study compared characteristics of the 58 subjects in whom new AAAs (≥3 cm) were detected with the 2,564 participants who did not have AAAs diagnosed at the 4-year followup; risk factor information on nonattendees, including the deceased, was also reported. Most of the detected AAAs were 3 to 3.4 cm (n=45), with a few in the 4- to 4.9-cm range (n=3). Nearly 3 percent (2.7%) of patients with AAA detected at the second screening had a positive family history of AAA compared with 6.0 percent of those without AAA. Less than 4 percent (3.4%) of participants with AAA detected at the second screening were black compared with 7.0 percent without AAA. Eighty-six percent of those with AAA detected were ever smokers (>100 cigarettes over a lifetime) compared with 74 percent in the group without AAA detected. Thirty-six percent of those with AAA detected were current smokers. Fifty-eight percent of those with AAA detected had any atherosclerosis compared with 42 percent without AAA detected. None of the 58 patients with AAA detected at rescreening were women. Mean age of those with AAA detected was similar to the mean age of those without AAA (67.3 and 66.0 years, respectively).

A univariate logistic model for predicting new AAA found the following characteristics to be significant: ever smoked (OR, 2.20 [95% CI, 1.04 to 4.66]), number of years smoked (OR, 1.26 [95% CI, 1.08 to 1.47]), current smoker at the time of initial screening (OR, 3.31 [95% CI, 1.92 to 5.72]), coronary artery disease (OR, 1.73 [95% CI, 1.03 to 2.91]), and any atherosclerosis, defined as coronary disease, cerebral vascular disease, or claudication (OR, 1.93 [95% CI, 1.14 to 3.28]; this composite factor resulted from subsequent reanalysis). A step-wise multivariate logistic model using significant factors from the univariate analysis resulted in three remaining significant factors: current smoker (OR, 3.09 [95% CI, 1.74 to 5.5]), coronary artery disease (OR, 1.81 [95% CI, 1.07 to 3.07]), and any atherosclerosis (OR, 1.97 [95% CI, 1.16 to 3.35]).

There was one AAA repair (likely from a false-negative result on initial screening) and no AAA deaths reported in any of the participants with a normal aorta, although this outcome came from national death records.

The smaller, fair-quality cohort study followed 223 patients selected from one of the Department of Veterans Affairs (VA) sites of the ADAM trial with normal aortas (<3 cm) on initial screening with yearly scans. The study found that 114 (63%) of these patients developed an aneurysm measuring larger than 3 cm at the mean 5.9-year followup, with the vast majority of detected AAAs being small (106/114 were 3.9 cm; 3/114 were >5 cm).[96] Multivariate logistic regression analysis did not identify any risk factors associated with the development of AAA. No AAA repairs, ruptures, or deaths were reported in those with initially normal aortas, although cause of death was obtained from death certificates only.

One fair-quality cohort study examined risk of AAA-related death in the 166 patients who developed AAA with rescreening (out of 4,308 with an initial normal scan who were rescreened) following an initial normal scan (<3.0 cm) and found no association between age group in this group and AAA death.[99]

KQ 2b. Does the Effect of Rescreening Vary Between Different Time Intervals?

In the five fair-quality and one good-quality prospective cohort studies[96-99,101,102] and one fair-quality case-control study,[100] screening occurred at various intervals after the initial normal scan, as follows: 3 months to annually,[98] annually,[96] at 5 years and 12 years,[102,103] every 2 years for up to 10 years or once after 5 years,[99] once at 4 years,[101] once at 3 to 5 years,[100] and every 2 years (**Appendix G Table 1**).[97] It is not possible to draw conclusions about the effect of screening frequency on health outcomes based on this small collection of heterogeneous studies with few, if any, reported AAA-related deaths.

KQ3. What Are the Harms Associated With One-Time and Repeated AAA Screening?

Summary of Results

All four large population-based screening RCTs (two fair-quality, two good-quality) provide information on operative mortality and number of AAA surgeries (**Table 1**).[13,14,94,95] Meta-analysis of available data at each time point (3 to 5 years, 6 to 7 years, 10 to 11 years, and 13 to 15 years) showed up to a doubling of risk for any AAA-related operation in the invited group, driven by more elective surgeries. The risk of emergency surgery was halved in the invited group compared with the control group. Thirty-day postoperative mortality after elective surgery was similar in screened and control groups, but was significantly reduced after emergency surgery in the screened group compared with the control group, for all time periods up to 10-year followup.

Five small observational studies (two cohort, one case-control, two cross-sectional) report conflicting results on the influence of AAA screening on quality of life and anxiety/depression measures. One study reported short-term decreases in quality of life at 12 months[104] in those who screened positive for AAA, while four studies showed no clinically important decline in quality of life measures in those who screened positive compared with unscreened controls.[13,95,105,128]

Three cohort studies[94,96,99] reported number of procedures, finding that relatively few (0.5%) of those with initially normal aortas will require elective or emergency surgery over 5 years (**Table 1**).

Study Details

One-Time Screening Harms

30-day postoperative mortality: all AAA surgeries, 3- to 5-year followup. Two of the four major screening RCTs (MASS, Chichester)[13,14] showed a statistically significant benefit in the invited group compared with the control group, while two trials showed no statistically significant difference at the 3- to 5-year followup period. Pooled data from the four trials using a random-effects model was performed, showing a point estimate of RR of 0.32 (95% CI, 0.21 to 0.48) (**Figure 6**) for 30-day mortality at 3 to 5 years. The fixed-effects model produced similar findings.

30-day postoperative mortality: all AAA surgeries, 7- to 15-year followup. MASS showed a similar decrease in 30-day mortality in the invited group at 7-, 10.1-, and 13.1-year followup (7-year RR, 0.32 [95% CI, 0.21 to 0.48], 10.1-year RR, 0.37 [95% CI, 0.25 to 0.54], 13.1-year RR, 0.46 [95% CI, 0.33 to 0.65]) (**Figure 6**).[90] Pooled results at 13 to 15 years, weighted mostly by the MASS results, showed a reduced 30-day postoperative mortality in the invited group (RR, 0.46 [95% CI, 0.34 to 0.63]).

30-day postoperative mortality: elective and emergency surgeries. Pooled data from MASS and the Western Australian trial showed no difference in 30-day mortality from elective surgery between the invited and control groups at 3- to 5-year followup (RR, 0.70 [95% CI, 0.35 to 1.41]) (**Figure 7**).[13] Results from the fixed-effects model yielded identical results. MASS reported 7- and 10-year outcomes, showing no difference in 30-day mortality from elective surgery between the invited and control groups.[89,90]

Pooled data from MASS and the Western Australian trial at 3- to 5-year followup showed reduced 30-day mortality from emergency surgery in the invited group (RR, 0.15 [95% CI, 0.07 to 0.32]) (**Figure 8**). Results from the fixed-effects model yielded similar results. MASS reported reduced 30-day mortality from emergency surgery at 7- and 10.1-year followup (7-year RR, 0.17 [95% CI, 0.09 to 0.31]; 10.1-year RR, 0.22 [95% CI, 0.13 to 0.36]).[89,90] MASS showed no difference in 30-day postoperative mortality between the groups at the 13.1-year followup.[129]

Number of AAA operations. In all trials, there were consistently more AAA-related operations in the invited group compared with the control group (**Table 1**). At 3 to 5 years, pooled analysis using a random-effects model from the four trials showed a doubling of any AAA-related operations in the screened group (RR, 2.16 [95% CI, 1.84 to 2.53]) (**Figure 9**). For every 1,000 individuals invited to be screened, five more underwent any AAA-related operation over the next 3 to 5 years (data not shown). Based on pooled data from three trials (MASS, Viborg, and Chichester), increased risk of AAA-related surgery in the screened group remained after 10 to 11 years, although the effect was somewhat diminished (RR, 1.57 [95% CI, 1.35 to 1.83]) (**Figure 9**). At 13 to 15 years, pooled data from three trials (Chichester, MASS, and Viborg) were similar to the 10- to 11-year time period (RR, 1.54 [95% CI, 1.38 to 1.72]). Sensitivity analysis using the fixed-effects model yielded similar results.

Number of elective operations. Elective operations were more common in the screened group in every trial at each of the followup time points (**Table 1**, **Figure 10**), with pooled relative risks for the various time points ranging from 3.25 (95% CI, 2.13 to 4.96) at 3 to 5 years to 2.07 (95% CI, 1.53 to 2.79) at 15 years. Heterogeneity was low at the 10- to 11-year and 13- to 15-year time periods. Based on pooled data at 3 to 5 years, 92 percent of all AAA operations in the screened group were elective compared with 64% of AAA-related operations in the control group (data not shown).

Number of emergency operations. Individual trial results varied, with most suggesting reduced emergency AAA operations in those invited for screening compared with controls over 5 to 15 years of followup (**Table 1**, **Figure 11**). Pooled results suggested that screening halved the risk of emergency surgery at 3 to 5 years (RR, 0.50 [95% CI, 0.29 to 0.86]), with some heterogeneity in individual RCT results (I^2=39%). The Western Australian trial alone reported a nonsignificant increased risk of emergency operations in the screened group at 3.6 years; this study also had a much higher proportion of elective surgeries (87%) in its control group compared with the other three trials (pooled percentage, 57%) (data not shown), which changed the relative effect of emergency operations between arms. By 13 to 15 years of followup, differences in emergency operations remained significant, and heterogeneity was low at this time point. Sensitivity analysis using the fixed-effects model yielded similar results.

Quality of life. One cohort, one augmented case-control, and one subsampling study were constructed from MASS,[13] Western Australian,[95] and Viborg[94] trial participants to address quality of life (data not shown). Two other observational comparisons were constructed from the Gloucestershire Aneurysm Screening program,[105] a regional Swedish screening program,[104] and one small screening study set in rural Australia.[128] The Viborg study was excluded, as it did not report baseline quality of life to allow adjusted comparisons among subgroups with and without AAA and with and without screening attendance.[94] The studies reported quality of life outcomes using different questionnaires, including the Short-form 36-item Health Survey (SF-36), Screen Quality of Life, European Quality of Life-Five Dimension (EuroQOL-5D), and the General Health Questionnaire (GHQ).[13,94,95,104,105,128] The SF-36 (range, 0 to 100) is a self-administered questionnaire evaluating eight domains: vitality, physical functioning, bodily pain, general health perceptions, physical role functioning, emotional role functioning, social role functioning, and mental health. The EuroQOL-5D (range, 0 to 100) is a generic measure of health status that provides a descriptive profile and a single index value that can be used in the clinical and economic evaluation of health care and in population health surveys. This self-administered questionnaire asks individuals to evaluate five dimensions: mobility, self-care, usual activities, pain/discomfort, and anxiety/depression. A lower number denotes poorer quality of life.

Questionnaires were administered at various time points, including prior to screening, after screening, or in selected subgroups of those with screen-detected AAA undergoing surgery or surveillance. Timing of questionnaires was no longer than 12 months after a specific event.

Prescreening quality of life. Baseline quality of life was gathered in 2009 from participants recruited to the Western Australian study during a specified period. Even prior to screening, those eventually found to have a small AAA had lower mean age-adjusted self-perceived general health on the EuroQOL-5D compared with those with normal aortas.[95] In the Gloucestershire Screening program, the GHQ was completed before screening and again after 1 month by 61 men with screen-detected AAA and 100 consecutively screened men with normal aortas.[105] No difference in overall score was seen in those with and without AAA, before or after screening, although anxiety decreased significantly in both groups 1 month after screening. Prior to undergoing ultrasound screening in a regional Swedish screening program, men and women completed the SF-36.[104] No baseline differences were seen in any SF-36 scale scores between men and women with AAA (n=27) and screen-negative age- and sex-matched controls. In the Australian study, the baseline SF-36 scores were not different between the men who subsequently screened positive or negative.[128]

Postscreening quality of life. Six weeks after screening, MASS compared depression, state anxiety, and quality of life using the SF-36, EQ-5D, Hospital Anxiety and Depression Scale, and Spielberger state/trait anxiety scales in a subset of those who screened positive for AAA, who screened negative, and who were not invited to screening. Those who screened negative showed no worse scores than unscreened controls, although those with screen-detected AAA had significantly worse anxiety, physical health, mental health, and self-rated health and health index quality of life scores than screen-negative participants. Even among those screening positive, anxiety and depression scores were well under clinical cutoffs, and quality of life scores were similar to those of unscreened controls. Longer-term data on the impact of screening on quality of life were not available, although physical and mental health scores and weighted health index scores in screen-positive patients undergoing surveillance or surgery tended to rebound after 3 months. In the Gloucestershire Screening program, no differences in overall GHQ scores were seen in those with and without AAA 1 month after screening, and anxiety was significantly reduced from baseline in both groups.[105] In the Western Australian trial, those with and without AAA had similarly sized, nonsignificant improvements in quality of life from baseline to 12 months after screening. In Swedish men and women, SF-36 scores were not different 12 months after screening in those with and without AAA; however, those with AAA showed significant decreases from baseline in physical functioning, social functioning, and mental health.[104] In the rural Australian study, SF-36 scores were not different 6 months after screening in those with and without AAA, but only the screen-negative group had a statistically significant improvement in the SF-36 dimensions of general health, social function, and freedom from bodily pain.[128] Small numbers make these results imprecise.

Rescreening Harms

No comparative data consider the effect of rescreening versus no rescreening on those without AAA on initial screening. Small cohort studies suggest that relatively few (0.5%) of those with initially normal aortas will require elective or emergency surgery over 5 years (**Table 3**). No studies examined quality of life outcomes for rescreening.

AAA surgeries. Three fair-quality cohort studies examined procedure rates in rescreened cohorts, showing that this rate varied from 0 to 0.5 percent (**Table 3**).[94,96,99] The largest of these three cohorts, with a 5-year followup, reported 17 elective and six emergency surgeries (out of 4,308 rescreened).[99]

30-day mortality. In the Hafez cohort study, six participants (out of 23 undergoing AAA operation [26.1%]) died within 30 days of surgery (**Table 4**).[99]

KQ 4. What Is the Effect of Pharmacotherapy Versus Placebo or Surgery (Open and EVAR) Versus Surveillance on Treatment-Relevant Intermediate Health Outcomes in an Asymptomatic Population With Small AAA Identified by Screening?

Summary of Results

Eight RCTs assessed the effects of early surgery versus surveillance (k=4)[106,108,113,115] and pharmacotherapy versus placebo (k=4)[116,118-120] in the treatment of patients with small AAA. In the two good-quality surgical trials comparing early open surgery with surveillance,[106,108] all-cause and AAA-related mortality at 5 years did not differ between the two approaches, although early open surgery significantly reduced the 5-year rupture rate (18 fewer AAA ruptures per 1,000 individuals treated with open surgery rather than surveillance). From available data, mortality effects after 8 and 12 years were unchanged;[41,109] very limited data evaluated subgroup differences, with no evidence of treatment differences in age- or aneurysmal diameter-specific subgroups. In the two fair-quality trials comparing early EVAR with surveillance,[113,115] shorter-term followup (at around 2 years) suggested no mortality or rupture benefit from early EVAR (leading to early cessation of both trials). A single good-quality drug trial found no significant effect on mortality or AAA growth rate after 2 years of beta-blocker use;[116] one good-quality and two fair-quality trials of different antibiotics used for 4 to 15 weeks also found no significant effect on mortality and found small, somewhat mixed effects on AAA growth rates, which are difficult to interpret.[118-120]

Study Details

Early Open Surgery Versus Surveillance

Two good-quality RCTs of early open surgery (UKSAT and ADAM),[106,108] conducted in the United Kingdom and the United States, enrolled a large number of patients (1,090 in UKSAT; 1,136 in ADAM) with small AAA (4.0 to 5.4 cm) and randomized them to early open surgery or surveillance (**Appendix H Table 1**). Both studies actively managed patients for a mean of approximately 5 years (4.6 years in UKSAT; 4.9 years in ADAM). In addition to 5-year followup at the end of active management, UKSAT reported results at 8 and 12 years.[109,130] Over 99 percent of patients were followed after 12 years in UKSAT, and approximately 86 percent in the ADAM trial after 5 years. The primary outcome for both trials was all-cause mortality, and secondary outcomes were cost (UKSAT) or AAA-related mortality reported by an independent outcomes committee (ADAM).

Important patient characteristics, such as age and smoking history, were comparable between the two studies, although UKSAT included a higher proportion of female patients (17.5% vs. 0.8%), lower rate of hypertension (39% vs. 56.4%) and ischemic heart disease (14% probable ischemic heart disease vs. 41.9% coronary disease), and fewer patients with diabetes (2.5% vs. 9.8%) (**Appendix H Table 2**). Mean AAA diameter at baseline was similar for the two studies (4.6 and 4.7 cm). For patients randomized to the early surgery group, procedures were undertaken 6 to 12 weeks after randomization, with 520 patients (92.4%) in UKSAT and 527 (92.6%) in the ADAM trial receiving procedures after a mean followup period of approximately 5 years. In the surveillance group, patients received an ultrasound every 3 to 6 months and were referred to surgery when the AAA diameter reached 5.5 cm, when the growth rate exceeded 0.7 cm in 6 months or 1 cm per year, or when they developed symptoms. By the end of 5-year followup, 321 (60.9%) patients in the UKSAT surveillance group and 349 (61.6%) in the ADAM surveillance group had undergone open surgical repair (**Table 5**).

The two RCTs of early open surgery versus surveillance (UKSAT, ADAM) reported outcome data at 5-year followup.[106,108] UKSAT, however, did not directly report AAA-related mortality. To determine this, we combined deaths from ruptured AAA data and 30-day operative mortality data. Although time-to-event data analyses were conducted in both trials, the effect estimates (i.e., HR) were available for pooling only for all-cause mortality.

The effects on all-cause mortality, AAA-related mortality, and rupture were consistent between the two trials (**Figure 12**, **Table 6**). At 5 years of followup, the ADAM trial reported similar findings between treatment groups in all-cause mortality (25.1% vs. 21.5%; HR, 1.21 [95% CI, 0.95 to 1.54]) and AAA-related mortality (3.0% vs. 2.6%; HR, 1.15 [95% CI, 0.56 to 2.31]).[106] UKSAT found an increase in all-cause mortality in those undergoing surveillance, though the difference was not significant (30.6% vs. 46.7%; HR, 0.91 [95% CI, 0.72 to 1.16]).[108] Pooling the two trials suggested no statistically significant difference in all-cause mortality (RR, 1.07 [95% CI, 0.91 to 1.25]) or AAA-related mortality (RR, 0.93 [95% CI, 0.64 to 1.37]) (**Figure 12**) between early open surgery and surveillance. Early open surgery did, however, significantly lower rupture risk (RR, 0.28 [95% CI, 0.13 to 0.62]), with 18 fewer AAA ruptures per 1,000 individuals treated with open surgery rather than surveillance after 5 years.

UKSAT further reported outcome data at 8 and 12 years of followup.[41,109] The results consistently showed no statistically significant difference in all-cause mortality (43.0% vs. 48.2% at 8 years; 64.3% vs. 66.8% at 12 years; RR, 0.96 [95% CI, 0.88 to 1.05]) and AAA-related mortality (9.6% vs. 7.0% at 8 years; 9.6% vs. 9.5% at 12 years; RR, 0.73 [95% CI, 0.49 to 1.09]) (**Table 6**). Early open surgery was reported to reduce the risk of rupture (1.8% vs. 4.3% at 8 years; 2.3% vs. 4.5% at 12 years). However, the relative magnitude of effect decreased over time due to a very similar, proportional increase in ruptured aneurysms in both arms, suggesting the reduced rupture benefit with open surgery occurs within the first 5 years (**Figure 12**).

The data for exploring heterogeneity across studies were very limited. Sensitivity analyses using reported HRs confirmed no statistically significant difference in all-cause mortality in early open surgery versus surveillance. The use of HRs, however, suggested higher heterogeneity (I^2=63.1%) than the use of risk ratios (I^2=21.4%), which might suggest a difference in the timing of deaths between the two trials (**Appendix K**). The use of alternative statistical models (random- vs. fixed-effects) did not show any significant change in 5-year effect estimates (**Appendix K**).

Early EVAR Versus Surveillance

Two medium-size, fair-quality, industry-funded RCTs (Comparison of Surveillance Versus Aortic Endografting for Small Aneurysm Repair [CAESAR],[113] Positive Impact of Endovascular Options for Treating Aneurysm Early [PIVOTAL][115]) were undertaken to evaluate the effect of early EVAR in patients with small aneurysms. CAESAR (N=360) measured the primary outcome of all-cause mortality and secondary outcomes of AAA-related mortality, rupture, growth, perioperative mortality, and conversion to open repair, while PIVOTAL (N=728) measured the primary outcome of AAA-related mortality and rupture and secondary outcomes of all-cause mortality and AAA-related mortality in smokers versus nonsmokers and conversion to open repair. Trials were conducted in the United States and Italy and randomized patients with small AAA (CAESAR, 4.1 to 5.4 cm; PIVOTAL, 4.0 to 5.0 cm) to undergo early EVAR versus surveillance (**Appendix H Table 2**). The CAESAR trial reported results at a median followup of 2.7 years, and the PIVOTAL trial reported results at a mean followup of 1.7 years. Notably, both RCTs conducted interim analyses and found that detection of meaningful difference in primary outcomes between EVAR and surveillance was unlikely if patient enrollment were to continue (i.e., futility).[113,115] Thus, both trials subsequently stopped recruiting patients early, but they completed scheduled followup in those who had already been enrolled. Likely due to early stopping of enrollment, the two studies did not adequately achieve balance between randomized arms in important prognostic factors, such as family history, sex, and diabetes.

While the mean age (70.5 vs. 68.9 years) and AAA diameter (4.45 vs. 4.72 cm) were similar between the trials, there was a higher proportion of smoking patients and patients with coronary artery disease in the PIVOTAL trial (91.0% vs. 55.3% and 55.4% vs. 39.2%, respectively) (**Appendix H Table 2**).[115] Both studies randomized patients to undergo EVAR within 30 days or to surveillance (**Appendix H Table 1**). Three hundred and twenty-two patients (88.9%) allocated to the early EVAR group underwent EVAR procedures in the PIVOTAL trial, and 171 (94.0%) in CAESAR (**Table 7**). In each of the studies, four patients received open surgery instead of EVAR in the early EVAR group. Patients in the surveillance group underwent assessment every 6 months and were offered EVAR when AAA diameter reached 5.5 cm, the growth rate exceeded 0.5 cm in 6 months or 1 cm per year, or they developed symptoms. Among patients randomized to surveillance, 71 (39.9%) in the CAESAR trial and 108 (30.1%) in the PIVOTAL trial received EVAR by the end of followup.

Both trials of early EVAR versus surveillance (CAESAR, PIVOTAL) reported the effect on all-cause mortality, AAA-related mortality, and rupture (**Tables 7** and **8**).[113,115] At the end of followup, early EVAR did not achieve a statistically significant reduction in the risk of all-cause mortality, AAA-related mortality, or rupture in either of the two RCTs compared with surveillance, but the number of events was generally small, with only zero to two events (AAA-related death or rupture) in each group reported in both studies (**Figure 13**, **Tables 7** and **8**). Both trials reported an all-cause mortality rate of approximately 4 percent, with similar results seen across treatment interventions (**Table 8**). Similarly, AAA-related mortality was found to be very similar across treatment arms and ranged from 0.3 to 0.6 percent (**Table 8**). Pooling data on all-cause and AAA-related mortality confirmed no difference in mortality between strategies, but pooled estimates were both in the direction of greater mortality with early EVAR (RR, 1.07 [95% CI, 0.62 to 1.86] for all-cause mortality; RR, 1.46 [95% CI, 0.24 to 8.94] for AAA-related mortality) (**Figure 13**). Both trials reported zero ruptures in the early EVAR group and low numbers in those receiving surveillance (0.3% and 1.1%) (**Table 8**). Pooling data on ruptures confirmed no difference in rupture rates between strategies (RR, 0.25 [95% CI, 0.03 to 2.26]) (**Figure 13**).

There was no statistically significant heterogeneity across the two trials (I^2=0% for all outcomes). Sensitivity analyses conducted with statistical models (random- vs. fixed-effects) did not show any significant change of the estimates (**Appendix K**).

Pharmacotherapy Versus Placebo

One good-quality and two fair-quality placebo-controlled parallel RCTs investigated the effectiveness of antibiotics (doxycycline, azithromycin, roxithromycin),[118-120] and one good-quality RCT investigated the effectiveness of the beta-blocker propranolol[116] compared with placebo for small AAA for the following outcomes: delay of AAA growth (primary outcome), all-cause mortality, AAA rupture, and surgery (**Appendix H Table 1**). These trials, conducted in Finland, Demark, Sweden, and Canada, recruited participants from vascular referral centers as well as community/population screening programs, had varying sample sizes with small antibiotic trials (34 to 211) and a single larger beta-blocker trial (N=552), and followed patients for 1.5 to 2.5 years. One study additionally reported results at 5 years of followup.[121] Only the doxycycline trial reported blinding outcome assessors.[118]

Important differences existed in patient characteristics across the four RCTs (**Appendix H Table 2**). Although the inclusion criteria were generally consistent, two trials included patients with AAA diameters of 3.0 to 5.0 cm,[116,120] one trial included AAA diameters of 3.0 to smaller than 5.5 cm,[118] and the other one included AAA diameters of 3.5 to 5.0 cm.[119] The four trials included patients of similar age (mean age, 68.4 to 72.5 years), but the proportion of female patients differed considerably between three trials (0% to 18.5%), and one trial exclusively enrolled men.[120] In three trials, about one third (34% to 40.0%) of patients had a smoking history, whereas the other trial included 59.5 percent of patients who were current or ever smokers.[120] The distribution of cardiovascular risk factors (e.g., the proportion of patients with hypertension, MI, or stroke) also differed across studies. Ultrasound measurements were performed using aortic anterior-posterior diameters in all trials, with three of the four trials using the larger of the axial or transverse measurement planes.[118-120] Only one trial[116] reported using outer-to-outer wall measurements, while the other three trials did not specify which wall measurements were used.

While three trials compared antibiotics with placebo, those antibiotics—including doxycycline, roxithromycin, and azithromycin—have different mechanisms (**Appendix H Table 1**).[118-120] The treatment duration ranged from 4 to 15 weeks. Patients were offered surgery when meeting surgical criteria, but these criteria were inadequately described in two trials.[118,119] The beta-blocker trial randomized patients to receive propranolol or placebo, with a target dose of between 80 and 120 mg twice daily, for a mean of 2.5 years.[116]

All three antibiotic trials reported all-cause mortality, the use of surgical procedures, and AAA growth rate (**Tables 9** and **10**).[118-120] We pooled the three trials in order to assess the overall effect of relatively short-term antibiotic use on all-cause mortality data. The pooled estimate suggested no effect of antibiotics above placebo on reducing all-cause mortality (RR, 0.92 [95% CI, 0.43 to 1.96]) (**Figure 14**). Despite the differences in patient characteristics and interventions, there was no statistically significant heterogeneity (I^2=0%). Pooling these trials suggested no statistically significant reduction in the use of surgical procedures for AAA in those taking antibiotics for 4 to 15 weeks compared with placebo (RR, 0.89 [95% CI, 0.51 to 1.55]) (**Appendix K**). The CIs for each trial were very wide, and no meaningful heterogeneity was found across studies (I^2=8.4%).

The reporting of AAA growth rate varied across the three trials (**Table 9**). Two trials reported median and interquartile range of annual growth rate,[118,119] whereas the other reported mean annual growth rate only.[120] The results were inconsistent across trials. One study showed no improvement with azithromycin over placebo (median, 2.2 vs. 2.2 mm per year; p=0.85).[119] Another study suggested a possible reduction in growth rate in patients using doxycycline versus placebo (median, 1.5 vs. 3.0 mm per year; no statistical testing reported).[118] Additionally, this study found that only one (7%) patient in the doxycycline group compared with five (41%) in the placebo group had an annual growth rate of 5 mm per year or more during 1.5 years of followup (p=0.06). In the third study, roxithromycin significantly reduced the growth rate compared with placebo at both 2 and 5 years of followup (mean, 1.56 vs. 2.75 mm per year at 2 years; p=0.02; 1.16 vs. 2.52 mm per year at 5 years; p=0.06);[120] nevertheless, the difference was too small to be clinically important, and care providers who measured AAA diameter were not blinded in those trials, which is a potential threat to the accuracy of measurement.

In the trial of propranolol versus placebo, there was no statistically significant reduction in all-cause mortality (12% vs. 9.6%; p=0.36), AAA-related mortality (0.7% vs. 0.7%; p=1.0), rupture (0.4% vs. 0.7%; p=0.25), or AAA growth rate (mean, 0.22 vs. 0.26 cm per year; p=0.11) (**Table 10**).[116]

Sensitivity analyses that compared random- versus fixed-effects models did not show any significant difference in the effect estimates (**Appendix K**).

KQ 4a. Does the Effect of Pharmacotherapy, Surgery, and Surveillance Differ Between Men and Women, Smaller and Larger Aneurysms, Smokers and Nonsmokers, Older and Younger Patients, Patients With and Without a Family History of AAA, Patients With and Without Diabetes, Patients With and Without COPD, and Patients of Different

Races/Ethnicities?

Summary of Results

At 5 years, two good-quality RCTs reported all-cause mortality by subgroups of age and AAA diameter, showing no significant differences.[106,108] One good-quality RCT reported no sex-specific subgroup difference in all-cause mortality.[108,103]

Study Details

Open Surgery Versus Surveillance: Subgroups by Sex, AAA Diameter, and Age

Sex. Only one trial of early open surgery versus surveillance reported all-cause mortality data by sex and found no significant sex-specific subgroup differences (adjusted HR for men, 0.9 [95% CI, 0.76 to 1.06]; adjusted HR for women, 0.89 [95% CI, 0.62 to 1.28]; p=0.76).[108,103] Through 12 years of followup, UKSAT found similar numbers of deaths in male and female participants in the early surgery group (8.0% in men vs. 8.4% in women) and slightly more deaths among women than men in the surveillance group (8.5% in men vs. 10.0% in women).

AAA diameter. When considering mortality by AAA diameter through 5 years of followup, both trials reported an increase in mortality as AAA diameter increased, with no significant differences between treatment groups. ADAM reported that 21.3 percent of those in the early surgery group and 16.2 percent of those in the surveillance group with an AAA diameter of 4.0 to 4.4 cm died (RR, 1.48 [95% CI, 0.92 to 2.38]).[106] Similarly, UKSAT reported more deaths in the early surgery group than in the surveillance group in those with AAAs measuring 4.0 to 4.4 cm (63 vs. 53 per 1,000 person-years; HR, 1.14; p=0.26).[108] In those with AAAs measuring 4.5 to 4.8 cm, there was no difference between treatment groups in UKSAT, and there were slightly more reported deaths in those receiving surgery in the ADAM trial (RR, 1.27 [95% CI, 0.81 to 1.99]). In both trials, there were no differences between treatment groups in those with AAAs measuring 5.0 to 5.4 cm (ADAM RR, 1.02 [95% CI, 0.71 to 1.47]; UKSAT HR, 0.79; p=0.26). We were able to conduct subgroup analyses across the two trials to examine whether the effect on all-cause mortality differed by AAA diameter. Our results confirmed what was reported above and showed no statistically significant difference in effects across the three AAA diameter subgroups (p=0.92 for interaction test) (**Appendix K**).

Age. In the ADAM trial, across all age groups, more deaths were seen in those receiving early open surgery, with an unsurprising increase in all-cause mortality as age increased (data not shown). This trend was slightly different in UKSAT, with more deaths in the surveillance group in those ages 60 to 71 years and more deaths in the early surgery group in those ages 72 to 76 years (data not shown). The subgroup data in UKSAT could imply a possible benefit of surgery in younger patients and a possible benefit of surveillance in older patients. These differences, however, were found to be nonsignificant, so the data should be interpreted with caution. In those ages 50 to 59 years in ADAM, there were no differences in mortality between those receiving early surgery and those undergoing surveillance (RR, 1.02 [95% CI, 0.38 to 2.73]).[106] Participants ages 60 to 69 years had 61 deaths in the early surgery group and 55 deaths in the surveillance group (RR, 1.34 [95% CI, 0.93 to 1.93]). In UKSAT, those ages 60 to 66 years had more deaths in the surveillance group than in the early surgery group (42 vs. 36 per 1,000 person-years; HR, 0.76; p=0.10). This trend was the same in those ages 67 to 71 years, with more deaths in those undergoing surveillance than early surgery (60 vs. 51 per 1,000 person-years; HR, 0.80; p=0.10).[108] In ADAM, at ages 70 to 79 years there were 74 deaths (27.3%) in those receiving surgery and 59 deaths (24.9%) in those receiving surveillance (RR, 1.10 [95% CI, 0.78 to 1.55]). In contrast, UKSAT reported more deaths in the early surgery group in those ages 72 to 76 years than in the surveillance group (72 vs. 48; HR, 1.25; p=0.10). Given that there was no overall effect on all-cause mortality, subgroup-specific effect modification is unlikely.[131]

As UKSAT and ADAM did not report results by comorbidity, family history, or race, no subgroup analyses are possible.

EVAR Versus Surveillance: Subgroups

Neither of the two trials comparing early EVAR surgery with surveillance reported data on subgroup effects.[113,115]

Pharmacotherapy Versus Surveillance: Subgroups

Of the three trials analyzing the effectiveness of antibiotics, only one reported data on subgroup effects by treatment arm (data not shown).[120] The roxithromycin trial (n=92) reported aneurysm expansion rates in each treatment group by AAA size through 2 years of followup. The results showed that roxithromycin was more effective at slowing aneurysm growth in both smaller and larger aneurysms, but not at significant levels. In aneurysms that were smaller than 3.65 cm at baseline, roxithromycin reduced aneurysm expansion compared with placebo, though not significantly (1.34 vs. 2.28 mm per year; p=0.17). This trend was similar to what was seen in aneurysms that were 3.65 cm or larger at baseline, with the difference again found to be not significant (1.76 vs. 3.27 mm per year; p=0.08).

The trial investigating the effectiveness of the beta-blocker propranolol did not report subgroup effects by treatment arm.[116]

KQ 5. What Harms Are Associated With Pharmacotherapy, EVAR and Early Surgery, and Surveillance in an Asymptomatic Population With Small AAA Identified by Screening?

Summary of Results

Both RCTs of early open surgery found a 50 percent increased risk of AAA-related surgical procedures in those randomized to early surgery instead of surveillance; for every 1,000 persons with small AAA managed with surveillance, 313 persons would avoid AAA-related surgery over 5 years.[106,108] For those requiring surgery in the surveillance arm, there was minimal difference in surgical complications after delayed open surgical repair compared with more immediate surgery (**Table 11**). No difference in 30-day operative or postoperative mortality was seen between early open surgery and delayed surgery; however, compared with immediate open surgery, 45 more individuals per 1,000 with small AAA undergoing delayed open surgery after surveillance would experience any complications, and two more would experience a major complication, particularly surgery-related MI. At least over the first 1 to 2 years after small AAA discovery, health perception/overall health was improved in those undergoing early open surgery, although there was no difference in overall quality of life (**Appendix I Table 1**).[107,132]

As expected, those with small AAA randomized to early EVAR more than doubled their risk of undergoing AAA-related surgery over the next several (1.5 to 2.5) years compared with those undergoing aneurysm surveillance (**Table 7**).[113,115] Between 484 and 582 out of every 1,000 persons with small AAA undergoing surveillance rather than early EVAR would be expected to avoid any AAA-related surgery during that time period. Delaying surgery until indicated after surveillance did not result in increased surgery-related harms, with some data suggesting better results in those undergoing delayed (as opposed to early) EVAR. Endoleaks were the most common complications after EVAR, occurring in 6 to 15 percent of participants in trials and one registry study. Differences in the risk of endoleaks between early and delayed EVAR were minimal, but favored delayed EVAR in one trial. Reinterventions over an unspecified time period were similar in early versus delayed EVAR in PIVOTAL, but were significantly increased after early EVAR in CAESAR, again favoring delayed EVAR (**Table 11**). As with early open surgery, short-term quality of life was significantly improved at 6 months in those undergoing early EVAR, but quality of life differences between approaches were not maintained after about 3 years of followup (**Appendix I Table 1**).[114]

Propanolol use more than doubled medication discontinuation or patient dropout compared with placebo (37.7% vs. 21.3%; p <0.0001 in the Propranolol Aneurysm Trial [PAT]; 60% vs. 40%; p-value not reported in the Danish trial), while relatively short-term antibiotic use had few reported harms or patient dropouts (0% to 2.4%) (**Table 11**).[116,117]

Study Details

Harms Associated With Early Open Surgery Versus Surveillance

Receipt of surgical procedures. At 5-year followup, approximately 93 percent of patients in the early open surgery group had received AAA repair in both trials, as opposed to approximately 61 percent in the surveillance group (**Appendix K, Table 5**).[106,108] The effect estimates were nearly identical between the two studies, and the pooled estimates (RR, 1.51 [95% CI, 1.44 to 1.59]) suggested that, at 5 years after randomization, 313 per 1,000 persons with small AAA managed with surveillance rather than open surgery would avoid any surgical procedure for AAA repair. By 12-year followup, UKSAT reported an additional 14 percent of the control group receiving AAA surgery. Nearly all surgeries (98% to 99%) were elective in both groups.

Operative mortality. At 5-year followup, the 30-day operative mortality in the early open surgery group of UKSAT was 5.8 percent (n=520) compared with 7.1 percent (n=321) in the surveillance group (**Table 11**).[108] In ADAM, 30-day operative mortality at 5 years was 2.0 percent (n=526) in the surgery group compared with 1.8 percent (n=340) in the surveillance group.[106] Pooling the data suggested no statistically significant difference in 30-day operative mortality between the two strategies (RR, 0.86 [95% CI, 0.54 to 1.36]) (**Figure 15**). In UKSAT, through 8 years of followup, each group had similar 30-day postoperative mortality rates compared with their respective 4.6-year followup rates. This suggests that delayed surgery did not alter 30-day postoperative mortality.

The results for postoperative mortality (adding in-hospital deaths after 30 days to 30-day operative mortality) were similar to 30-day mortality, with pooled results suggesting no statistically significant difference between the two strategies (RR, 0.86 [95% CI, 0.54 to 1.37]) (**Appendix K**).

Surgical complications. The ADAM trial, but not UKSAT, reported 30-day readmissions and (nonfatal) complications associated with AAA repair in both groups (**Table 11**).[106] Findings were limited by relatively few participants and low individual event rates. Patients in the early open surgery group tended toward a slightly higher rate of 30-day readmissions (20.5% vs. 16.5%), but had a significantly lower risk of any surgical complications (52.3% vs. 56.8%; p=0.026). Nonetheless, the event rate for total major complications was higher in the surveillance group (4.4% to 7.9%), with a significantly higher risk of surgery-related MI reported (1.0% vs. 3.8%; p=0.0051).

Quality of life. Both UKSAT and ADAM reported quality of life, although only UKSAT reported numerical data (**Appendix I Table 1**). UKSAT reported change in quality of life, measured by the Medical Outcomes Study 20-item Short-form Health Survey, 1 year after randomization.[132] This questionnaire measures multiple domains of patient health, including physical functioning, role functioning, social functioning, metal health, current health perception, and bodily pain. The total score ranges from 0 to 100, with a higher score indicating better health. In patients of both groups, quality of life appeared to decrease 1 year after randomization across all domains (1- to 6-point decrease), except that health perception was improved in the early surgery group (approximate 6-point increase). There was no statistically significant difference in the change of quality of life from baseline between early open surgery and surveillance in most domains, although patients in the early surgery group had better health perception after 1 year. The difference in mean change of health perception was 6.7 points (95% CI, 3.41 to 9.99) between groups, suggesting a clinically meaningful improvement.[133]

The ADAM trial measured patients' quality of life using the SF-36, and collected data every 6 months until the end of followup.[107] Patients were followed for 3.5 to 8 years (mean, 4.9 years), and approximately 86 percent of patients completed followup. The study analyzed change in quality of life over time using a repeated-measures model and adjusting for baseline measurements. The authors reported a statistically significant decrease in all SF-36 subscales over time for the entire population (p<0.001). Although numerical values are not reported, they are presented graphically. No difference, however, was found between the early repair group and the surveillance group in all SF-36 subscales, except that the early repair group had statistically higher general health scores (p<0.001). This difference was due mainly to significantly higher scores during time points between 6 months and 2 years (p<0.05).

The ADAM trial also reported rates of impotence among participants.[107] In a repeated-measures analysis, there was a statistically higher risk of developing impotence over time in patients with early repair than those undergoing surveillance (p<0.03). The statistically significant difference occurred between 18 months and 4 years. No numerical values were reported.

Harms Associated With Early EVAR Versus Surveillance

Two registry studies assessing EVAR reported harms data,[122,123] in addition to the two RCTs of early EVAR versus surveillance described in KQ 4 (**Appendix H Table 1**).[113,115] The two fair-quality registry studies, conducted in Australia (Australian Safety and Efficacy Register of New Interventional Procedures-Surgical [ASERNIP-S])[122] and Europe (European Collaborators on Stent/Graft Techniques for Aortic Aneurysm Repair [EUROSTAR]),[123] prospectively collected data from patients with AAA who underwent EVAR. The ASERNIP-S study collected perioperative and intermediate outcome data associated with EVAR from Australia's national audit and included more than 90 percent of procedures performed. The EUROSTAR study documented all patients undergoing EVAR with commercially available devices approved in continental Europe. Both studies reported results according to the size of AAA at baseline, thus allowing the assessment of harms associated with EVAR in patients with small AAA. The ASERNIP-S study enrolled 478 patients with small AAA (≤5.5 cm), and the EUROSTAR study included 4,392 patients, of which 1,962 had small AAA (4.0 to 5.4 cm). The median length of followup was 3.2 years (interquartile range, 2.4 to 3.7 years) in ASERNIP-S and approximately 1.7 years (range, 1 month to 8 years) in EUROSTAR.

Use of surgical procedures. After 1.7 years of followup, endovascular procedures were undertaken in more than 89 percent of patients in the early EVAR group in the PIVOTAL trial and 96 percent at 2.5 years in the CAESAR trial (**Table 7**).[113,115] In the surveillance group, EVAR was undertaken in 31 percent of patients in PIVOTAL and 48 percent in CAESAR. Both studies found a statistically significant increase in the receipt of surgical procedures in the early EVAR group, with a greater increase suggested in PIVOTAL than in CAESAR (pooled RR, 2.41 [95% CI, 1.68 to 3.45]) (**Appendix K**). Using the pooled estimate, 549 of every 1,000 individuals with small AAA managed with surveillance rather than early EVAR would avoid any surgical procedure for AAA in 1.5 to 2.5 years. Given that the two trials had quite different estimates (reflected in high heterogeneity when pooled), the estimate for the number avoiding surgery could range from a low of 484 per 1,000 (as seen in CAESAR) to a high of 582 per 1,000 (as seen in PIVOTAL).

Operative mortality. In both trials, 30-day operative mortality after EVAR was rare; only one patient died in the early EVAR group in each trial (0.3% in PIVOTAL; 0.6% in CAESAR), while one patient undergoing repair in the surveillance group of PIVOTAL died and none died in CAESAR (**Table 11**).[113,115] Because of this low event rate, the CI of the pooled estimates was very wide (RR, 0.63 [95% CI, 0.08 to 5.12]) (**Figure 16**), but these results do not suggest increased operative mortality from delaying surgery through surveillance. In the registry studies, the 30-day mortality among those receiving EVAR was slightly higher (1.1% in ASERNIP-S; 1.6% in EUROSTAR).[122,123] The difference was likely due to the fact that registry studies included higher-risk patients or to other differences in community practice.

Complications. The reporting of complications and the time periods assessed differed considerably across the four studies (two RCTs and two registry studies) (**Table 11**).[113,115,122,123] In PIVOTAL, approximately 4 percent of patients required reinterventions over an unspecified time period in both groups, suggesting no difference in reinterventions for those undergoing early versus delayed surgery after surveillance.[115] Endoleaks were the most frequent 30-day complication, occurring in 10 to 12 percent of patients receiving EVAR, but were not different between those undergoing early versus delayed EVAR (after surveillance). Other 30-day complications, including endograft or peripheral thromboses, wound infections, and systemic complications, occurred in about 15 percent of EVAR recipients, with no difference in early versus delayed surgery.

In the CAESAR study, the percentage of patients with any morbidity was significantly higher in the early EVAR group than the surveillance group at 30 days (18% vs. 6%; p<0.01) and after 30 days to 2.5 years (19% vs. 5%; p<0.01) (**Table 11**).[113] Although the groups did not differ in the number of major adverse events early or late in the study, the early EVAR group had significantly more endoleaks after 30 days to 1 year (12% vs. 2.8%; p=0.028) and significantly more secondary procedures than the surveillance group (5.7% vs. 0%; p=0.03).

Both the ASERNIP-S and EUROSTAR registry studies reported mortality and complications after EVAR in participants with small AAA (30-day postoperative mortality in ASERNIP-S, timing not reported in EUROSTAR), with much less detail in EUROSTAR (**Table 11**).[122,123] The rate of systemic complication (defined as cardiac, pulmonary, renal, cerebral, or gastrointestinal complications) was similar: 13.4 percent in ASERNIP-S and 12.0 percent in EUROSTAR. The rate of device and procedural complications, however, appeared much higher in ASERNIP-S (10.7% within 30 days of surgery) than EUROSTAR (2.9%, unclear timeframe). The two registry studies additionally reported complications at longer followup (median of 3.2 years in ASERNIP-S and 1.7 years in EUROSTAR). In the ASERNIP-S study, 97 (20.3%) patients had endoleaks during followup (28% requiring reintervention). EUROSTAR compared the cumulative probability of various types of endoleaks (i.e., type I proximal, type I distal, type II, and type III), but incomplete reporting did not allow us to determine the cumulative probability of having an endoleak. The cumulative probability of conversion to open surgery was 6.6 percent.[123]

Quality of life. Data from one trial (CAESAR) compared short-term (6 months) and longer-term (mean, 3 years [SD, 1.2 years]) quality of life in those with small AAA randomized to early EVAR versus surveillance[114] (**Appendix I Table 1**). Compared with baseline, overall quality of life improved at 6 months in patients receiving EVAR (**Figure 16**), with larger benefits in the mental health summary score than the physical health summary score. In contrast, quality of life decreased slightly from baseline to 6 months in the surveillance group, thereby favoring early EVAR for all of these measures. By the end of followup, both groups showed decreases in quality of life from baseline, and none of these quality of life summary scores differed between groups.

Harms Associated With Pharmacotherapy

In addition to the four RCTs described in KQ 4,[106,108,113,115] one additional RCT of propranolol versus placebo provided harms data only.[117] This RCT randomized 54 patients with small AAA to receive either 40 mg of propranolol twice daily (n=30) or placebo (n=24) for 2 years (**Appendix H Table 1**). A large proportion of patients (60% in propranolol group vs. 29% in placebo group) dropped out of the study, mainly because of adverse events. Thus, while the trial was ineligible for assessment of benefits because of significant loss to followup, it provided useful data about harms associated with propranolol in the treatment of AAA.

Two trials assessing propranolol reported data about adverse effects that led to medication discontinuation[116] or patient dropout.[117] Both studies suggested that propranolol at least doubled patient discontinuation of medications or dropout from the study (37.7% vs. 21.3%; p <0.0001 in PAT;[116] 60% vs. 40%; p-value not reported in the Danish trial[117]) (**Table 11**). In PAT, propranolol was associated with a higher rate of fatigue, shortness of breath, and bradycardia or atrioventricular block, and was possibly associated with higher risk of heart failure.[116] Because of the small sample size in the Danish trial, adverse events were generally very low. More adverse events, however, occurred in patients receiving propranolol across all adverse event categories.[117]

The three antibiotic trials reported medication discontinuation and associated side effects (**Table 11**).[118-120] Generally, results suggested that these antibiotics used over 4 to 15 weeks were not associated with a significant increase of harms. In the trial of doxycycline, two patients (one with doxycycline, one with placebo) out of 32 total participants discontinued medication because of allergic reactions.[118] The trial of roxithromycin reported no medication discontinuation.[120] Two patients in the treatment group and two in the placebo group, out of a total of 247 participants, discontinued medication in the trial of azithromycin due to gastrointestinal symptoms, diarrhea, and arthralgia. Additionally, one patient in the treatment group discontinued medication due to allergic reaction, but this was found to be caused by an antihypertension medication. The trial of azithromycin also reported that 21 patients (13 in the treatment group and eight in the control group; p=0.37) had side effects. Details about the side effects, however, were unknown. Two of the three antibiotic trials[119,120] reported a need for surgery in each group; however, due to a small number of events overall, conclusions are limited.

Chapter 4. Discussion

Summary of Review Findings

Table 12 presents a summary of evidence for each KQ in order, which we briefly discuss next.

Direct Evidence on Mortality Benefit of Screening

Based on four large, population-based screening trials with up to 15 years of followup,[13-16] our current meta-analysis confirms the conclusions of prior meta-analyses that there is convincing direct evidence that offering screening to men age 65 years and older decreases AAA-related mortality by approximately 50 percent over 13 to 15 years.[134-136] Little controversy exists about the presence and magnitude of this AAA-related mortality benefit incurred with screening in men age 65 years and older, although the same is not true for all-cause mortality.[134,137] While the most recent meta-analysis,[138] which included the latest followup from MASS at 13.1 years,[129] found a statistically significant reduction in all-cause mortality (fixed effect OR, 0.973 [95% CI, 0.950 to 0.997]), it combined mortality outcomes reported across followup times ranging from 3.6 to 15 years. Our meta-analysis used a random-effects model measuring risk ratio and found no statistically significant reduction in all-cause mortality; sensitivity analyses using ORs yielded similar point estimates to the most recent other meta-analysis.[138]

Expecting a meaningful reduction in all-cause mortality with one-time screening might be considered optimistic, given that AAA prevalence at age 65 years is around 4 percent, large AAA prevalence (>5 cm) is much less common (approximately 0.5%), and ruptures are rare (0.1% to 0.6% at 5 years). Even if the AAA-related mortality benefit from screening is close to a 50 percent risk reduction, a major effect on all-cause mortality might be unachievable since many large AAAs at risk for rupture will be found in older patients who have competing causes of mortality and comorbidities that limit their surgical candidacy.

A more detailed analysis of 7-year findings from MASS suggests that AAA-related mortality curves diverge at 1 year after screening, with life-years gained in the invited group increasing at a constant rate over the next 6 years.[89] One-time screening in men age 65 years and older was very cost-effective (<$30,000 U.S. per life-year gained) at 7 years.

Harms of Screening

With direct evidence of an overall and sustained AAA-related mortality benefit, specific screening-related harms are most relevant to patient-centered decisionmaking. Not surprisingly, screening leads to more elective AAA repairs but fewer AAA ruptures and less deaths due to emergency repairs. Making conclusions about psychological harms is more challenging; quality of life studies are small, largely (4 out of 5) case-control studies, and quite heterogeneous, with different study populations, scales, and followup periods. One study showed that the decreased quality of life in the screen-positive group (compared with the screen-negative group) at 6 weeks did not persist.[13] Other studies showed prescreening versus postscreening quality of life to be lower or no different.[89,104,105] One study showed that having small AAA followed by surveillance was associated with a lower quality of life compared with control.[98]

Direct and Indirect Evidence for Screening in Subgroups

Women

The Chichester trial provides the only direct evidence about the effect of AAA screening on health outcomes in women.[25] Among 9,342 women ages 65 to 80 years, the AAA rupture rate in the invited and control groups was similarly low at 5 years (approximately 0.06% in both groups) and 10 years (0.19% and 0.21%, respectively). No sex-specific effect on AAA-related mortality was seen at 5 years. However, these findings are not definitive due to the relatively modest numbers of women studied and the sex-specific differences in the natural history of AAA demonstrated: AAA prevalence in women was six times rarer than in men (affecting power), and more AAA-related deaths occurred after age 80 years in women than in men (70% in women compared with <50% in men).[25]

A number of reports have found that women experience a consistent, three- to four-fold higher risk of AAA rupture than men.[51,54,58,139] Three studies provide additional evidence that AAA rupture occurs at a smaller diameter in women than in men.[54,58,140] In a cohort of 2,257 patients, including subjects from UKSAT and the U.K. Aneurysm Study, the mean AAA diameter preceding rupture was 6.0 cm (standard error, 1.4) in men compared with 5.0 cm (standard error, 0.8) in women (p=0.001).[54] In a Canadian cohort (n=476), women were four times more likely to experience AAA rupture than men at diameters between 5.0 and 5.9 cm (95% CI, 1.2 to 13.0; p<0.001).[58] The annual rupture rate at diameters larger than 6.0 cm was 14.1 percent for men and 22.3 percent for women. In a small Finnish study of 166 participants, 24 percent of women experienced AAA rupture at a diameter of smaller than 5.5 cm compared with 5 percent of men.[140]

A greater risk for large (≥5.0 cm) AAA rupture and for rupture at smaller diameters among women could reflect the greater proportional dilation of the normal female aorta to the 5.5 cm diameter threshold that triggers surgical intervention. A Canadian study of 129 subjects affirmed that AAAs of equal diameter represent a greater proportional dilation in women.[141] Another factor suggested to contribute to greater risk for women is anatomical complexity associated with aneurysm repair[142] due to smaller access vessels in women.[48,143] One report suggests that EVAR delivery sheaths are relatively large for the female population.[139]

Data from a large ultrasound study found that female sex was significantly associated with smaller mean infrarenal aortic diameter (-0.14 cm) among those with normal aortic diameters after multivariable adjustment; absolute differences of 0.1 cm in infrarenal aortic diameter were equivalent to larger changes in other independent variables, such as age (29 years).[144]

From a population perspective, while the risk of AAA rupture is relatively higher in women than men, the absolute risk of AAA-related death in women, even in female smokers, is quite a bit lower than in men, largely due to the lower prevalence of AAA. In a prospective U.K. cohort study of 1.2 million women (median age, 55 years) followed for a period of 12 years, 330 current smokers (0.028%) and 164 female never-smokers (0.014%) died of AAA.[145] A recent Swedish screening study in 5,140 women showed that the overall prevalence of AAA in women was 0.5 percent and was 0.8 percent and 2.1 percent, respectively, in female ever-smokers and current smokers.[146]

Age

Age at initial screening could be important for understanding the risks and benefits demonstrated in the four major trials. The oldest men recruited to the trials ranged from an initial age of 73 to 80 years. The prevalence of AAA was higher in the two trials with older mean/median ages (Chichester and Western Australian) than in the two trials with younger enrollment ages (7% to 7.7% vs. 4%). Offering screening to an older population would theoretically result in greater benefit due to a higher yield of larger AAAs (>5 cm) that could be repaired to prevent rupture; however, only one of these trials demonstrated a reduction in AAA-related mortality with screening. Competing risks and limited suitability for surgical repair could offset the higher prevalence with older age.

Two trials reporting age-specific subgroups found no age-specific differences in the effects of screening on AAA-related or all-cause mortality.[15,16] After 13 years, older men (ages 66 to 73 years) had a similar relative risk reduction for AAA-related mortality as younger men ages 64 to 65 years.[15] After 3.6 years, no AAA-related mortality benefit was seen in the Western Australian trial, either overall or in age-specific subgroups (75 years and older vs. 65 to 74 years). While not suggesting age-specific differences, these data are limited by overall power, distribution and range of ages compared, and number of studies examining these subgroup issues.

Family History

Family history remains one of the stronger individual risk factors after adjusting for age, sex, and smoking status (**Table 13**). In a large study (n=3,183 AAA cases; 15,943 controls) using Swedish population-based registries, researchers confirmed a doubling of AAA risk among those with one or more first-degree relatives with AAA, regardless of the sex of the index case or relative, and whether or not they also had comorbid conditions.[46] Siblings appear to be a particularly relevant group, with a reported frequency of AAA of 11 percent,[147] 6 percent,[148] and 4 percent[149] in recent studies; female siblings appear to have much lower relative and absolute risk than male siblings. Among 10,012 female volunteers, the highest prevalence of screen-detected AAA was among women age 75 years and older (1.5%) and those with indications of heart disease (i.e., prior MI, coronary revascularization, or other cardiac surgery) (2.0%).[12] Among 7,657 women age 65 years and older, the 464 women who were ever-smokers with heart disease (6%) had an AAA prevalence of 3.4 percent, while the few women who were ever-smokers with heart disease and a family history (n=31 [0.4% of women age 65 years and older]) had a prevalence of 6.6 percent.[12] At least in women, these data suggest that family history alone would be insufficient to identify women to screen, as would smoking status. It is not clear how much family history would contribute to screening effectiveness in men beyond current recommendations.

Comorbidity

A single screening trial (Viborg) reported AAA prevalence and AAA-related mortality outcomes in trial participants with and without six AAA-associated comorbidities.[125] Longer-term[93] or risk-factor specific[125] analyses from this trial were not available at the time of the prior USPSTF recommendation.[1] Based on the presence of one or more hospital discharge diagnoses (COPD, MI, hypertension, ischemic heart disease, peripheral artery disease, stroke, or transient ischemic attack), about one quarter (26.5%) of invited and control participants were considered high-risk at baseline, and these individuals had almost half (88/191) of all AAAs detected on screening. However, high-risk screening based on this approach would involve a tradeoff; it would screen 73 percent fewer patients but prevent only half of AAA deaths compared with a mass screening strategy. After a mean observation period of 5.9 years, AAA-related mortality was reduced by 8.4 deaths per 1,000 high-risk patients invited to screening (compared with no screening) and 3.7 deaths per 1,000 lower-risk patients. These data suggest a clearly superior benefit in those at higher risk status, presumably based on higher prevalence of AAA. Longer-term outcomes (13 years) from the same trial show a consistent relative risk reduction after screening in high-risk and lower-risk groups but a larger absolute AAA-mortality benefit in the high-risk group than the low-risk group. This study is limited in that the risk factor collection and analysis were done after trial randomization and risk-stratified comparisons represent subgroup analyses that do not conform to criteria for high-quality subgroup findings (i.e., those based on a significant treatment-by-group interaction or on subgroups that were balanced in the randomization process).[93] Also, because comorbidities were derived from hospital discharge summaries, these high-risk participants were likely a select subgroup of the population, thereby creating bias against the projected yield from high-risk targeted screening.

Risk Scoring

Although we found minimal direct evidence addressing subgroups in our systematic review, determining the most effective and efficient approaches to population-based AAA screening remains an important issue. In response to the 2005 USPSTF recommendation for a selective screening approach targeting male ever-smokers ages 65 to 75 years, concerns have been voiced about missed opportunities to prevent AAA rupture, particularly in women, younger nonsmoking men, and those with a family history of AAA. Specifically, critics note the substantial rupture rate and number of AAA-related deaths that occur in women (at least 33% of ruptured AAA hospitalizations and 41% of AAA-related deaths), while nonsmokers account for about 22% of AAA-related deaths.[150-152] Perhaps a different high-risk approach (beyond smoking, age, and male sex) could identify a group with increased prevalence of AAA, and thereby be more effective and equally efficient. However, many higher-risk individuals have known comorbidities that could affect eligibility and/or complications associated with surgical treatment that could compromise the ability to attend surveillance. Thus, several studies have evaluated the yield and value of high-risk approaches, targeting those with existing or suspected cardiovascular conditions[153,154] and/or COPD.[125] As described above, investigators from the Viborg study determined that limiting screening to men with COPD and/or other CVD would reduce the number of individuals screened by 73 percent but miss more than half (52%) of AAAs in men ages 65 to 73 years.[125] Screening in a cardiac clinic referral population resulted in a high (9.5%) prevalence of AAA (≥3 cm), all which were detected in patients older than age 60 years, who were four times more likely to be male and three times more likely to have ischemic heart disease.[153] No consideration was given to whether those with AAA were suitable for surgical management. In a separate cardiology clinic setting, a similarly high prevalence (9.9%) of newly detected AAA was seen in male attendees ages 65 to 75 years, which was much higher than (5.4%) in men of the same age from the community.[154] Ten percent of AAAs were large enough (≥5 cm) to consider surgery, but not all (one of four large AAAs) were eligible for open surgery or EVAR, and one of three patients with a repaired AAA had a complicated recovery due to comorbidity. In a retrospective study of individuals referred to a vascular laboratory, patients with screen-detected AAA were older (mean age, 72.8 years) and more likely to have competing comorbidities compared with those detected in screening trials; as a consequence, these patients were also less likely to undergo elective repair (21.5%) or full surveillance (48%), often due to poor health.[155] Less than half (47.5%) were alive at the mean followup of 7.5 years (SD, 2.8), with more than half (56.8%) of deaths due to cardiac or cerebrovascular disease; one third (32.6%) due to cancer, COPD, or other nonvascular causes; 10.6 percent due to other vascular causes; and less than one in 10 (8.5%) related to the AAA (3.2% aortic rupture, 4.2% postoperative, 1.1% aortic dissection).

Using large-scale cohort data and/or population-based models, investigators have examined whether different targeted approaches could detect more clinically significant AAA with the same or better efficiency than the 2005 USPSTF recommended approach. One early effort developed and tested a novel multivariable risk factor score using data from the Western Australian screening trial. Results suggested that 50 percent of the male population would need to be screened to detect 75 percent of aneurysms measuring 4 cm or larger, while screening male ever-smokers would detect 87 percent of these aneurysms but require screening about two thirds of men.[156] From this early study, authors concluded that mass screening remained preferable to selective screening, but they acknowledged that risk-prediction models based on better data might change this conclusion.

More recently, investigators developed and validated a novel scoring tool to predict prevalent AAA using demographic and medical history data from 3.1 million individuals who volunteered for community-based ultrasound screening.[157] This study sample was different from the group currently recommended by the USPSTF for screening, as it was predominantly female (65%) and younger (20% age 55 years and younger, 34% ages 55 to 64 years). Prevalent AAA (infrarenal abdominal aortic diameter ≥3 cm) was detected in 0.77% of screened subjects (n=23,446), who were mainly male (79%), white (91%), and current or past smokers (80%). Among all age groups, the highest proportion of AAA detected was in those ages 65 to 74 years (44%), with more than half in persons outside the current USPSTF screening age range (i.e., 20% younger than age 65 years and 36% age 75 years and older). The majority (73%) of detected AAAs were small (3 to 4 cm), with a minority (17%) measuring from 4 to 5 cm, and just 10 percent considered large (≥5 cm); size distribution did not appear to vary with age. Based on multivariable analysis, male sex, age older than 60 years, and smoking at least one half pack per day for more than 10 years each independently increased the odds of any AAA five-fold (**Table 13**). Beyond confirming the strong and independent value of risk factors used to target screening (male sex, older age, smoking history) among those with an increased AAA prevalence, these data point out the contribution of family history of AAA and more detailed smoking history (pack-years). The analyses point out some protective factors that modify AAA risk (e.g., years since quitting smoking) or are associated with reduced AAA prevalence (e.g., nonwhite race/ethnicity, diet, exercise, diabetes). These risk factors were converted to scores based on their relative weights, which added up to a total AAA risk score ranging from 0 to 100.

The best predictive model for presence of AAA incorporated age, sex, detailed smoking history, race/ethnicity, cardiovascular risk factors and comorbidities, family history of AAA, diet, exercise, and body mass index. In the development subset of the cohort, this model discriminated well between those with and without AAA (area under the curve [AUC], 0.893). When tested in the remaining validation subset of the cohort, discrimination was diminished (AUC, 0.842) but calibration was very high (r^2=0.98 for the association between predicted and observed probability of having an AAA, within each total risk score).

To further focus on detecting clinically significant AAA, the same investigators developed and validated a new model for predicting the presence of large AAA ($\geq$5 cm) using a similar study sample from the same voluntary screening population, but also including those age 85 years and older.[158] There were 2,430 individuals (0.08% of all persons screened) with an AAA of 5 cm or larger; 84.4 percent of those with large AAAs were male and 83% were ever-smokers. Few (18%) large aneurysms occurred in those younger than age 65 years, with the remainder evenly divided between those ages 65 to 74 years (41%) and age 75 years and older (41%). About one third (36.3%) of the large AAAs in this cohort occurred in the 207,493 male ever-smokers ages 65 to 75 years who would be recommended for screening using the 2005 USPSTF recommendation. As **Table 13** illustrates, some factors (such as male sex and older age) are even more strongly associated with large AAA than with any AAA.

In order to compare the potential effect of various risk-based screening strategies in the United States, these same investigators modified their initial risk prediction models to include only risk factors available in National Health and Nutrition Examination Survey data to estimate the prevalence of any AAA or large AAA in the U.S. population.[157,158] Using these data on estimated prevalence, the authors then simulated the yield and screening requirements of various risk-based screening strategies.

These simulations suggest that the 2005 USPSTF approach is reasonably effective and relatively efficient for detecting any AAA or large AAA compared with universal screening. Current screening data also support the USPSTF approach, with recent studies reporting that more than 80 percent of AAAs were found in ever-smokers.[11,159,160] The current USPSTF recommendation is estimated to detect 29.5 percent of an estimated 1.1 million prevalent AAAs in the U.S. population, requiring 20 screenings per AAA found. For any large AAA, the simulated yield of the 2005 USPSTF approach would detect 33.7 percent of an estimated 120,810 large AAAs, requiring 168 screenings per large AAA detected. The simulated yield and requirements of different screening approaches based on risk scores could potentially detect more AAAs of any size than the USPSTF strategy (from 42.3% to 66.5% of estimated prevalent AAAs) at about the same efficiency, or could be more effective at detecting large AAAs (from 45.8% to 84.2% of estimated large AAAs) at increased efficiency (67 to 156 screenings per AAA detected).

However, in these simulated strategies, the age distribution of screen-detected large AAA also tends to shift to the older age groups (>75 years). As has been demonstrated in other studies,[155] cases detected in older or more ill individuals may be less likely to be eligible for surgical repair or may have worse perioperative morbidity/mortality and long-term survival than cases detected in large screening trials, thus potentially reducing the expected health benefit from these types of risk-based screening strategies.

While intriguing, these findings require some caveats. First and foremost, by simulating yield, these data cannot represent health outcomes due to incompletely capturing issues around treatment eligibility and harms. Second, these risk models are both derived from the same cohort and are validated only internally; either would require external validation in a completely separate cohort before clinical application could be considered.[161] This is particularly true since the internally-derived risk factor profile was used to project the prevalence of AAA in the general population, and thus the model may be more optimistic than if it were assessed against empirically documented AAAs. Also, as the development and validation cohort was based on individuals who were primarily self-referred, the self-reported risk factors in this cohort may not be comparable with the U.S. population to whom it was applied. Third, the modified risk model used in the simulations excluded some strong contributors to the risk score in the original model, particularly family history of AAA. Although the AUC of the modified model was reported to be almost as good as the initial model, AUC is an insensitive measure of model differences since it is based solely on rankings.[162] Authors did not report other comparisons of the two models. Finally, all of these modeled data are cross-sectional and presume that prevalent AAA in individuals older than the USPSTF screening range are undetected and equally important to detect (i.e., as amenable to preventive benefit from clinical intervention) as those in younger adults; similarly, the simulations presume that prevalent AAAs in those younger than age 65 years are important to detect before recommended screening would commence at age 65 years (or are in groups who are never recommended to receive AAA screening).

Nonetheless, these interesting data should encourage further investigation and consideration of more targeted risk strategies for detecting and treating AAA early to prevent AAA-related mortality and morbidity. In particular, a risk prediction emphasis on detecting larger aneurysms could address in part the important issue of potential overdiagnosis in older adults (who might have smaller aneurysms that would never progress enough to require intervention). Further research in this area should be a high priority since these studies suggest important, feasible strategies that could improve AAA screening recommendations overall and for underserved groups, including women, younger high-risk adults, and older healthy adults. Moreover, it would be extremely useful to have more robust models for assessing the value and requirements of risk-based screening approaches that address various surveillance and treatment approaches, competing risks and contraindications to treatment, and rescreening across a broader population group.

Recent Decline in AAA Prevalence

Recent epidemiologic evidence from population-based screening programs in Europe and New Zealand demonstrate a substantial decline in AAA prevalence in men age 65 years and older over the past two decades, with current AAA prevalence reported at 1.5 to 1.7 percent (AAA

≥3cm).[11,17-19] There have not been any similar epidemiologic reports from the United States, likely because screening uptake is low, which makes it difficult to estimate the true prevalence in the population of men age 65 years and older.[163] Declining smoking rates could largely account for this observed decline,[164,165] though there is likely also a contribution from declining atherosclerotic disease due to aggressive management of hypertension and hyperlipidemia with statins.[11,146] This decline in prevalence must be considered carefully in estimating the yield from mass versus targeted screening approaches and certainly favors a more targeted approach (i.e., ever-smokers) similar to that which the USPSTF previously recommended. One recent retrospective chart review from the Northern California VA (2007 to 2011) of male veteran ever-smokers ages 65 to 75 years with a mean age of 71.5 years (N=9,751) reported a prevalence of AAA of 3 cm or larger of 7.1 percent, but there were more smaller aneurysms detected than previously reported (only 6.6% of AAAs detected were ≥5.5 cm compared with 12% in MASS).[166] This suggests that even if the overall prevalence of AAA were declining in the United States as it is in other countries, the risk of AAA in ever-smokers may continue to remain high, with a shift toward smaller aneurysms. No single risk factor other than age, sex, or smoking history is as strong of a predictor of AAA, thereby making a multiple risk factor approach appealing once a validated risk score is available.

National/International Guidelines

Differing international guidelines reflect variations in the interpretation of direct and indirect evidence on AAA screening in subgroups (**Appendix J**). While most guidelines have some consensus on the starting age of 65 years for one-time screening, the upper age limit is unspecified in most recommendations. In those specifying an upper age limit, most recommend stopping at age 75 years (USPSTF, American College of Cardiology [ACC], Canadian Society for Vascular Surgery), while one organization recommends stopping at age 85 years (Society for Vascular Surgery).[1,24,167-169] The USPSTF 2005[1] and ACC[168] guidelines specify smoking as a risk factor for targeted screening, while others incorporate family history of AAA into the definition of a target population.[24,168,169] Several guidelines recommend screening in high-risk women, where high-risk is defined as having CVD risk factors and/or a family history of AAA,[24,167,169] whereas other organizations, such as the ACC and USPSTF, do not recommend screening women.[1,168] Guidance on the screening interval for ultrasound surveillance is generally based on AAA size on initial screening but varies widely; generally, larger aneurysms (>4.0 to 4.5 cm) are rechecked every 6 to 12 months, with 1 to 3 years for smaller aneurysms.[1,24,167-169]

Treatment Studies for Small AAA

The AAA-related mortality benefit in screening trials was achieved through immediately referring large AAAs (>5.5 cm) for appropriate surgical treatment, while monitoring smaller aneurysms with repeat ultrasounds every 3 to 12 months followed by surgical referral for rapid growth or reaching large AAA size over about 5 years. An important opportunity for increasing the expected net benefit from current screening programs could come from potential improvements in the surveillance and surgical management of small AAAs, particularly since these are much more common than larger aneurysms.

Two major, good-quality RCTs provide robust assessment of the benefits and harms of early open surgery compared with surveillance of small AAA in populations applicable to clinical practice.[106,102] There is strong evidence that early open surgery compared with surveillance does not reduce all-cause or AAA-related mortality, although it reduces 5-year risk of rupture (18 fewer AAA ruptures per 1,000 individuals with small AAA treated with early open surgery rather than surveillance). Early open surgery resulted in 50 percent more surgical procedures (313 more surgeries per 1,000 persons with small AAA). There was no difference in postoperative or 30-day operative mortality among those undergoing early versus delayed open surgical repair, but those undergoing delayed surgical repair may have slightly more total complications (45 per 1,000 persons undergoing delayed rather than immediate repair) or major complications (2 per 1,000 persons), particularly postoperative MI. Early surgery generally does not improve patients' overall quality of life, although health perception may be improved in the first 1 to 2 years. In one trial, early open surgery increased the risk of impotence over the first several years.

Two moderate-sized, fair-quality trials assessed the benefits and harms of early EVAR versus surveillance in patients with small AAA who are applicable to clinical practice.[113,115] These two trials are limited by relatively short-term followup and a small number of events due to early stopping for reaching futility (i.e., the statistical impossibility of treatment showing a benefit). Although point estimates are imprecise, available data suggest no difference in the risk of all-cause mortality, AAA-related mortality, or AAA rupture with surveillance instead of early EVAR. Those in the surveillance arm were able to avoid an estimated 549 surgeries (range, 484 to 582) per 1,000 individuals with small AAA managed through surveillance rather than early EVAR, and surgical outcomes (30-day operative mortality or complications) for delayed surgery after surveillance showed no difference when compared with early EVAR. Early EVAR was associated with improved quality of life, at least over the short term, but may also result in more short- and longer-term device-related endoleaks. Two moderately-sized, fair-quality registry studies found two to three times higher 30-day operative mortality with EVAR than in these trials (1.1% to 1.6% vs. ≤0.5%), suggesting further caution in treating small aneurysms with early EVAR based on available evidence.

Pharmacological treatment may minimize aneurysm progression, but current evidence is too limited in quality and in numbers of patients and types of treatments studied to make many firm conclusions. There is adequate evidence only for propranolol, which has little to no effect on AAA growth rate, all-cause mortality, AAA-related mortality, and rupture. It is poorly tolerated, with significantly increased adverse effects and frequent discontinuation of treatment. In contrast, studies of antibiotics generally do not show many adverse effects, but these studies cannot demonstrate a clear finding on AAA growth rate, all-cause mortality, AAA-related mortality, and rupture because of heterogeneous patient populations, short-term administration (4 to 15 weeks), differences in outcome reporting, and small numbers of events.

Generally, current evidence reviewed here or by others does not support the treatment of small AAA with early open surgery, early EVAR,[170] or pharmacotherapy.[171] In our review, patients identified with small AAA appeared to experience some decline in quality of life during followup, with any differences due to management strategies primarily limited to short-term effects favoring intervention. It is possible that patient reassurance may alleviate concerns leading to decreased quality of life, but this was beyond the scope of our review.

Rescreening

There remains controversy regarding the yield of rescreening after a normal initial screening. Some authors have used incident AAA and growth rates to advocate rescreening at 2-, 4-, or 5-year intervals.[98-100] Six of our included studies[96,98-102] report AAA growth in normal aortas (2.5 to 3 cm); the largest study[99] (4,308 participants) and one other included study[98] showed a growth rate of 1.7 to 1.8 mm per year for a median 4- to 5-year followup in those with aortas measuring 2.5 to 2.9 cm. Five trials show a rare AAA-related mortality (0% to 0.56%) at 5- to 10-year followup with various rescreening intervals in those with aortas measuring 2.5 to 2.9 cm on initial scan.[96,97,99,101,102] A larger analysis from the ADAM study[101] showed that current smoking, coronary disease, and any atherosclerosis were predictive of incident AAA at the 4-year rescreening interval, but in this study of over 5,000 veterans, AAA-related mortality was zero. Again, many of these newly detected (incident) AAAs (incident rate, 2.2 [95% CI, 1.7 to 2.8] at 4 years) will be small (only 3 of 58 new AAAs were 4 to 4.9 cm and none were ≥5 cm). While it may be tempting to use these growth rates and incident AAAs to make decisions about rescreening frequency, most incident AAAs are small and may not have clinical consequence.

Incidental AAA on Computed Tomography Examination

Incidental AAAs are aneurysms identified when the abdomen is imaged for other reasons, such as colorectal cancer screening.[172] One systematic review of 17 studies found that 0.9 percent of subjects undergoing computed tomography (CT) colonography screening had a finding of incidental AAA.[173] We did not locate any studies that followed subjects with negative incidental AAA findings on CT scan to determine the negative predictive value of no incidental finding.

Two studies, however, report that findings of positive incidental AAA are not well documented or followed up.[174,175] In a retrospective cohort of 191 patients with incidental AAA found by ultrasound, magnetic resonance imaging, or CT with a median observation time of 4.4 years, 29.3 percent of subjects had no followup imaging of their aneurysm,[174] and only 26 percent of those who were inpatients had discharge summaries mentioning the finding. Another retrospective cohort found that in 61.4 percent of 83 incidental AAAs, there was no documentation that the primary care physician was aware of the results in the electronic medical record within 3 months of the CT scan.[175] Using a multivariable regression model, the study found that subjects with incidental AAA not receiving radiological monitoring for 1 year were significantly more likely to die (HR, 2.99) compared with subjects receiving recommended radiological monitoring; this finding was independent of age, baseline AAA diameter, care setting, and patient morbidity.

Based on these limited data, previous CT scanning could not be presumed to substitute for recommended AAA screening, since it is not clear how completely CT scans for other purposes identify incidental AAA. Further, when incidental AAAs are identified, they may not be as effectively surveyed as those detected in a structured screening program.

Limitations Due to Our Approach

Our approach might be limited by several factors, including a reliance on English-language literature only, a requirement for RCTs or large cohort studies for screening and treatment benefits, and a requirement that studies meet the USPSTF's fair- or good-quality criteria.[86] Similarly, as the focus of this systematic review was to update a previous USPSTF review,[44] some issues, such as risk assessment, incidental AAA detection on CT screening for other purposes, and possible sex differences in the risk of rupture at a specific aortic diameter, were addressed as part of the introduction or discussion but not systematically reviewed.

Limitations Due to the Evidence Base

Population Screening Issues

The four large population-based screening trials, while robust in numbers, almost exclusively represent a population of older Caucasian men. There is no direct evidence examining AAA-related mortality benefit in any subpopulations other than women and older men; the single screening study in women was underpowered to detect differences in health outcomes. While populations of smokers, those with a family history of AAA, and those with CVD represent groups with higher risk of AAA, there is no direct evidence examining the health outcomes resulting from screening these populations. Likewise, there is no direct evidence about high- and low-risk approaches to screening.

Repeat Screening Trials

The cohort studies examining AAA growth and mortality were not adequately powered to detect differences in health outcomes afforded by screening, and the body of rescreening literature is heterogeneous, with various surveillance intervals and treatment protocols.

Harms of Screening

The literature examining quality of life and psychological harms of screening comprised a heterogeneous group of cohort, case-control, and observational studies derived from subsets of larger trials using different instruments and followup periods, making long-term harms difficult to quantify. There were no studies examining AAA-specific quality of life instruments.

Treatment Studies

Inconsistent definitions of treatment-related morbidity across surgical treatment studies complicate their interpretation and limit their use in syntheses. Most nonsurgical treatment studies were conducted using relatively small, short-term studies of selected populations, with limited variability (or undocumented variability) in important potential effect modifiers (such as smoking, sex, age, and comorbidity). Women were underrepresented in the ADAM, CAESAR, and pharmacotherapy trials. No RCTs examined the benefits of several potentially promising pharmacologic treatments for small AAA, such as statins, ACE inhibitors, or better tolerated beta-blockers. Few treatment studies are designed to adequately assess health outcomes. Focus on AAA growth rate could be a useful intermediate outcome if future studies more consistently report AAA growth using the same metrics at the same time points and with some quality assurance of measurements, in addition to other important bias minimization tools, such as blinding of outcomes assessors.

Emerging Issues/Next Steps

Screening

Because the etiology of AAA is not fully understood, independent risk factors for AAA development as well as factors influencing AAA growth remain to be defined, including the role of genetic markers in AAA development. While a few hypotheses have been posited to explain AAA growth, none has been confirmed by clinical studies designed to address these hypotheses. Investigation of additional mechanisms and possible interactions among the mechanisms may be warranted. Targeted screening approaches continue to be an area of debate in the literature; accurate identification of high-risk populations who could survive and benefit from surgery remains a challenge.

There is some emerging interest in exploring the potential effects of AAA screening on CVD mortality by identifying those at increased risk for atherosclerotic coronary disease and ischemic stroke.[176,177] MASS reported ischemic heart disease–related deaths in screened and unscreened groups, showing no difference at 13 years, thereby questioning whether AAA screening has such effects.[129]

Treatment

There is a need to further explore alternative strategies to reduce AAA growth, such as antibiotics, statins, or other novel pharmacologic agents. Interventions to address modifiable risk factors (particularly smoking) may be worth considering in reducing AAA growth. Effective smoking cessation strategies may improve the care of patients with small AAA.

Future Research

Screening

The yield of targeted screening approaches in populations with CVD, peripheral vascular disease, and family history of AAA, as well as the yield of rescreening, will continue to be debated using simulated models until large screening RCTs with sufficient power and a decade or more of followup can confirm such benefit. In the absence of such a trial, a risk-scoring approach with associated health outcomes will need to be developed and validated in the U.S.

population.

There is one in-progress RCT on screening: the Viborg Vascular screening trial, which is evaluating the effectiveness of combined screening for AAA (ultrasound), peripheral artery disease (ankle–brachial index), and hypertension in 50,000 men ages 65 to 74 years recruited from a central Denmark national registry (**Appendix C**).[178] Enrollment began in October 2008 and ended in 2010, with planned followup at 3.5, 10, and 15 years. For those who screen positive for AAA or peripheral artery disease, trained nurses will provide advice on exercise, low-fat diet, and smoking cessation, and medical management with statins and aspirin will be initiated. Annual surveillance for AAA and peripheral artery disease will be provided, and those with AAAs measuring 5.0 cm or larger will be referred for vascular surgery. The trial's primary outcome is all-cause mortality ascertained from national death registries; secondary outcomes include cardiovascular mortality, AAA-related mortality, AAA prevalence and progression, health-related quality of life, and cost-effectiveness.

Finally, there is one prospective cohort screening trial in Oslo recruiting 1,500 men age 65 years, with a primary outcome of AAA prevalence/incidence and a secondary outcome of peripheral artery disease incidence in participants with AAA over an 18-year followup period, with an estimated completion date of 2029 (**Appendix C**).

Treatment

More efforts are needed to examine the effect of pharmacotherapy for the treatment of small AAA in large, high-quality RCTs with longer followup and measurement of health outcomes (AAA-related and all-cause mortality). While a number of observational studies have demonstrated the effect of statins on growth,[179] RCTs measuring health outcomes are needed.

Currently, there are seven ongoing RCTs examining pharmacotherapy effects on small AAA (3 to 5 or 5.5 cm): two small angiotensin receptor blocker trials measuring growth or AAA incidence, one ACE inhibitor trial, two small trials of anti-inflammatory medications, and two doxycycline trials (**Appendix C**). The primary outcome in most trials is aneurysmal growth. These trials are all small and underpowered to detect differences in health outcomes.

Conclusions

The following new literature has been published since the last systematic review performed to support the 2005 USPSTF recommendation:[44] longer-term followup from four population-based RCTs confirming the AAA-related mortality benefit afforded from screening; one new simulation study examining high-risk versus low-risk targeted approaches;[125] and a few internally-validated simulation models assessing the effectiveness and efficiency of risk-scoring systems. Treatment literature in this interim period has confirmed the lack of benefit from open surgery or EVAR for small AAA compared with surveillance and no evidence of benefit of pharmacotherapy for small AAA, thereby making the detection of small AAA more problematic.

References

1.   U.S. Preventive Services Task Force. Screening for abdominal aortic aneurysm: recommendation statement. *Ann Intern Med.* 2005;142(3):198-202. PMID: 15684208.
2.   Johns Hopkins Medicine. Abdominal Aneurysm. Baltimore, MD: The Johns Hopkins University; 2013. Accessed at http://www.hopkinsmedicine.org/vascular/conditions/Abdominal on 7 January 2013.
3.   VascularWeb®. Abdominal Aortic Aneurysm. Chicago: Society for Vascular Surgery; 2011. Accessed at http://www.vascularweb.org/vascularhealth/Pages/abdominal-aortic-aneurysm.aspx?PF=1 on 7 January 2013.
4.   Moll FL, Powell JT, Fraedrich G, et al. Management of abdominal aortic aneurysms: clinical practice guidelines of the European Society for Vascular Surgery. *Eur J Vasc Endovasc Surg.* 2011;41(Suppl 1):S1-58. PMID: 21215940.
5.   Wanhainen A. How to define an abdominal aortic aneurysm—influence on epidemiology and clinical practice. *Scand J Surg.* 2008;97(2):105-9. PMID: 18575024.
6.   Wanhainen A, Svensjo S, Mani K. Screening for abdominal aortic aneurysm—areas where information is still inadequate. *Scand J Surg.* 2008;97(2):131-5. PMID: 18575030.
7.   Cornuz J, Sidoti PC, Tevaearai H, et al. Risk factors for asymptomatic abdominal aortic aneurysm: systematic review and meta-analysis of population-based screening studies. *Eur J Public Health.* 2004;14(4):343-9. PMID: 15542867.
8.   Jamrozik K, Norman PE, Spencer CA, et al. Screening for abdominal aortic aneurysm: lessons from a population-based study. *Med J Aust.* 2000;173(7):345-50. PMID: 11062788.
9.   Conway AM, Malkawi AH, Hinchliffe RJ, et al. First-year results of a national abdominal aortic aneurysm screening programme in a single centre. *Br J Surg.* 2012;99(1):73-7. PMID: 21928466.
10. Schermerhorn M, Zwolak R, Velazquez O, et al. Ultrasound screening for abdominal aortic aneurysm in medicare beneficiaries. *Ann Vasc Surg.* 2008;22(1):16-24. PMID: 18055170.
11. Svensjo S, Bjorck M, Gurtelschmid M, et al. Low prevalence of abdominal aortic aneurysm among 65-year-old Swedish men indicates a change in the epidemiology of the disease. *Circulation.* 2011;124(10):1118-23. PMID: 21844079.
12. Derubertis BG, Trocciola SM, Ryer EJ, et al. Abdominal aortic aneurysm in women: prevalence, risk factors, and implications for screening. *J Vasc Surg.* 2007;46(4):630-5. PMID: 17903646.
13. Ashton HA, Buxton MJ, Day NE, et al. The Multicentre Aneurysm Screening Study (MASS) into the effect of abdominal aortic aneurysm screening on mortality in men: a randomised controlled trial. *Lancet.* 2002;360(9345):1531-9. PMID: 12443589.
14. Scott RA, Wilson NM, Ashton HA, et al. Influence of screening on the incidence of ruptured abdominal aortic aneurysm: 5-year results of a randomized controlled study. *Br J Surg.* 1995;82(8):1066-70. PMID: 7648155.
15. Lindholt JS, Juul S, Fasting H, et al. Screening for abdominal aortic aneurysms: single centre randomised controlled trial. *BMJ.* 2005;330(7494):750. PMID: 15757960.
16. Norman PE, Jamrozik K, Lawrence-Brown MM, et al. Population based randomised controlled trial on impact of screening on mortality from abdominal aortic aneurysm. *BMJ.* 2004;329(7477):1259. PMID: 15545293.
17. Darwood R, Earnshaw JJ, Turton G, et al. Twenty-year review of abdominal aortic

aneurysm screening in men in the county of Gloucestershire, United Kingdom. *J Vasc Surg*. 2012;56(1):8-13. PMID: 22503187.

18. National Health Service. NHS Abdominal Aortic Aneurysm Screening Programme: 2011–12 Summary. London: National Health Service; 2013.

19. Sandiford P, Mosquera D, Bramley D. Trends in incidence and mortality from abdominal aortic aneurysm in New Zealand. *Br J Surg*. 2011;98(5): 645-51. PMID: 21381003.

20. Vardulaki KA, Walker NM, Day NE, et al. Quantifying the risks of hypertension, age, sex and smoking in patients with abdominal aortic aneurysm. *Br J Surg*. 2000;87(2):195-200. PMID: 10671927.

21. Duncan JL, Wolf B, Nichols DM, et al. Screening for abdominal aortic aneurysm in a geographically isolated area. *Br J Surg*. 2005;92(8):984-8. PMID: 16034847.

22. Palombo D, Lucertini G, Pane B, et al. District-based abdominal aortic aneurysm screening in population aged 65 years and older. *J Cardiovasc Surg*. 2010;51(6):777-82. PMID: 21124273.

23. Bush RL, Lin PH, Lumsden AB. Endovascular management of abdominal aortic aneurysms. *J Cardiovasc Surg*. 2003;44(4):527-34. PMID: 14627225.

24. Chaikof EL, Brewster DC, Dalman RL, et al. The care of patients with an abdominal aortic aneurysm: the Society for Vascular Surgery practice guidelines. *J Vasc Surg*. 2009;50(4 Suppl):S2-49. PMID: 19786250.

25. Scott RA, Bridgewater SG, Ashton HA. Randomized clinical trial of screening for abdominal aortic aneurysm in women. *Br J Surg*. 2002;89(3):283-5. PMID: 11872050.

26. Agency for Healthcare Research and Quality. Healthcare Cost and Utilization Project: Nationwide Inpatient Sample Data Set. Report No. 43. Rockville, MD: Agency for Healthcare Research and Quality; 2006.

27. Lederle FA, Nelson DB, Joseph AM. Smokers' relative risk for aortic aneurysm compared with other smoking-related diseases: a systematic review. *J Vasc Surg*. 2003;38(2):329-34. PMID: 12891116.

28. Stolle K, Berges A, Lietz M, et al. Cigarette smoke enhances abdominal aortic aneurysm formation in angiotensin II-treated apolipoprotein E-deficient mice. *Toxicol Lett*. 2010;199(3):403-9. PMID: 20937366.

29. Laughlin GA, Allison MA, Jensky NE, et al. Abdominal aortic diameter and vascular atherosclerosis: the Multi-Ethnic Study of Atherosclerosis. *Eur J Vasc Endovasc Surg*. 2011;41(4):481-7. PMID: 21236707.

30. Trollope AF, Golledge J. Angiopoietins, abdominal aortic aneurysm and atherosclerosis. *Atherosclerosis*. 2011;214(2):237-43. PMID: 20832800.

31. Abdul-Hussien H, Hanemaaijer R, Kleemann R, et al. The pathophysiology of abdominal aortic aneurysm growth: corresponding and discordant inflammatory and proteolytic processes in abdominal aortic and popliteal artery aneurysms. *J Vasc Surg*. 2010;51(6):1479-87. PMID: 20488324.

32. Kaneko H, Anzai T, Morisawa M, et al. Resveratrol prevents the development of abdominal aortic aneurysm through attenuation of inflammation, oxidative stress, and neovascularization. *Atherosclerosis*. 2011;217(2):350-7. PMID: 21530968.

33. Thompson AR, Drenos F, Hafez H, et al. Candidate gene association studies in abdominal aortic aneurysm disease: a review and meta-analysis. *Eur J Vasc Endovasc Surg*. 2008;35(1):19-30. PMID: 17920311.

34. Nordon IM, Hinchliffe RJ, Holt PJ, et al. Review of current theories for abdominal aortic

aneurysm pathogenesis. *Vascular.* 2009;17(5):253-63. PMID: 19769804.

35. Collin J, Heather B, Walton J. Growth rates of subclinical abdominal aortic aneurysms— implications for review and rescreening programmes. *Eur J Vasc Surg.* 1991;5(2):141-4. PMID: 2037085.

36. Powell JT, Sweeting MJ, Brown LC, et al. Systematic review and meta-analysis of growth rates of small abdominal aortic aneurysms. *Br J Surg.* 2011;98(5):609-18. PMID: 21412998.

37. Wilmink AB, Quick CR. Epidemiology and potential for prevention of abdominal aortic aneurysm. *Br J Surg.* 1998;85(2):155-62. PMID: 9501808.

38. Reed WW, Hallett JW Jr, Damiano MA, et al. Learning from the last ultrasound. A population-based study of patients with abdominal aortic aneurysm. *Arch Intern Med.* 1997;157(18):2064-8. PMID: 9382661.

39. Scott RA, Tisi PV, Ashton HA, et al. Abdominal aortic aneurysm rupture rates: a 7-year follow-up of the entire abdominal aortic aneurysm population detected by screening. *J Vasc Surg.* 1998;28(1):124-8. PMID: 9685138.

40. Conway KP, Byrne J, Townsend M, et al. Prognosis of patients turned down for conventional abdominal aortic aneurysm repair in the endovascular and sonographic era: Szilagyi revisited? *J Vasc Surg.* 2001;33(4):752-7. PMID: 11296328.

41. Powell JT. Long-term outcomes of immediate repair compared with surveillance of small abdominal aortic aneurysms. *N Engl J Med.* 2002 May 9;346(19):1445-52. PMID: 12000814.

42. Wilmink AB, Hubbard CS, Day NE, et al. The incidence of small abdominal aortic aneurysms and the change in normal infrarenal aortic diameter: implications for screening. *Eur J Vasc Endovasc Surg.* 2001;21(2):165-70. PMID: 11237791.

43. Thompson AR, Cooper JA, Ashton HA, et al. Growth rates of small abdominal aortic aneurysms correlate with clinical events. *Br J Surg.* 2010;97(1):37-44. PMID: 20013940.

44. Fleming C, Whitlock EP, Beil TL, et al. Screening for abdominal aortic aneurysm: a best-evidence systematic review for the U.S. Preventive Services Task Force. *Ann Intern Med.* 2005;142(3):203-11. PMID: 15684209.

45. van Vlijmen-van Keulen CJ, Pals G, Rauwerda JA. Familial abdominal aortic aneurysm: a systematic review of a genetic background. *Eur J Vasc Endovasc Surg.* 2002;24(2):105-16. PMID: 12389231.

46. Larsson E, Granath F, Swedenborg J, et al. A population-based case-control study of the familial risk of abdominal aortic aneurysm. *J Vasc Surg.* 2009;49(1):47-50. PMID: 19028058.

47. MacSweeney ST, O'Meara M, Alexander C, et al. High prevalence of unsuspected abdominal aortic aneurysm in patients with confirmed symptomatic peripheral or cerebral arterial disease. *Br J Surg.* 1993;80(5):582-4. PMID: 8518892.

48. Lederle FA, Johnson GR, Wilson SE, et al. Relationship of age, gender, race, and body size to infrarenal aortic diameter. The Aneurysm Detection and Management (ADAM) Veterans Affairs Cooperative Study Investigators. *J Vasc Surg.* 1997;26(4):595-601. PMID: 9357459.

49. Helgadottir A, Thorleifsson G, Magnusson KP, et al. The same sequence variant on 9p21 associates with myocardial infarction, abdominal aortic aneurysm and intracranial aneurysm. *Nat Genet.* 2008;40(2):217-24. PMID: 18176561.

50. Lederle FA, Johnson GR, Wilson SE, et al. The aneurysm detection and management study

screening program: validation cohort and final results. Aneurysm Detection and Management Veterans Affairs Cooperative Study Investigators. *Arch Intern Med.* 2000;160(10):1425-30. PMID: 10826454.

51. Sweeting MJ, Thompson SG, Brown LC, et al. Meta-analysis of individual patient data to examine factors affecting growth and rupture of small abdominal aortic aneurysms. *Br J Surg.* 2012;99(5):655-65. PMID: 22389113.

52. Lederle FA, Johnson GR, Wilson SE, et al. Rupture rate of large abdominal aortic aneurysms in patients refusing or unfit for elective repair. *JAMA.* 2002;287(22):2968-72. PMID: 12052126.

53. Darling RC, Messina CR, Brewster DC, et al. Autopsy study of unoperated abdominal aortic aneurysms. The case for early resection. *Circulation.* 1977;56(3 Suppl):ii161-4. PMID: 884821.

54. Brown LC, Powell JT. Risk factors for aneurysm rupture in patients kept under ultrasound surveillance. UK Small Aneurysm Trial Participants. *Ann Surg.* 1999;230(3):289-96. PMID: 10493476.

55. Cronenwett JL, Murphy TF, Zelenock GB, et al. Actuarial analysis of variables associated with rupture of small abdominal aortic aneurysms. *Surgery.* 1985;98(3):472-83. PMID: 3898453.

56. Fillinger MF, Raghavan ML, Marra SP, et al. In vivo analysis of mechanical wall stress and abdominal aortic aneurysm rupture risk. *J Vasc Surg.* 2002;36(3):589-97. PMID: 12218986.

57. Venkatasubramaniam AK, Fagan MJ, Mehta T, et al. A comparative study of aortic wall stress using finite element analysis for ruptured and non-ruptured abdominal aortic aneurysms. *Eur J Vasc Endovasc Surg.* 2004;28(2):168-76. PMID: 15234698.

58. Brown PM, Zelt DT, Sobolev B. The risk of rupture in untreated aneurysms: the impact of size, gender, and expansion rate. *J Vasc Surg.* 2003;37(2):280-4. PMID: 12563196.

59. Lederle FA, Walker JM, Reinke DB. Selective screening for abdominal aortic aneurysms with physical examination and ultrasound. *Arch Intern Med.* 1988;148(8):1753-6. PMID: 3041938.

60. Lindholt JS, Vammen S, Juul S, et al. The validity of ultrasonographic scanning as screening method for abdominal aortic aneurysm. *Eur J Vasc Endovasc Surg.* 1999;17(6):472-5. PMID: 10375481.

61. Costantino TG, Bruno EC, Handly N, et al. Accuracy of emergency medicine ultrasound in the evaluation of abdominal aortic aneurysm. *J Emerg Med.* 2005;29(4):455-60. PMID: 16243207.

62. Tayal VS, Graf CD, Gibbs MA. Prospective study of accuracy and outcome of emergency ultrasound for abdominal aortic aneurysm over two years. *Acad Emerg Med.* 2003;10(8):867-71. PMID: 12896888.

63. Quill DS, Colgan MP, Sumner DS. Ultrasonic screening for the detection of abdominal aortic aneurysms. *Surg Clin North Am.* 1989;69(4):713-20. PMID: 2501880.

64. Graeve AH, Carpenter CM, Wicks JD, et al. Discordance in the sizing of abdominal aortic aneurysm and its significance. *Am J Surg.* 1982;144(6):627-34. PMID: 7149120.

65. Long A, Rouet L, Lindholt JS, et al. Measuring the maximum diameter of native abdominal aortic aneurysms: review and critical analysis. *Eur J Vasc Endovasc Surg.* 2012;43(5):515-24. PMID: 22336051.

66. Norman PE, Jamrozik K, Lawrence-Brown MM, et al. Western Australian randomized

controlled trial of screening for abdominal aortic aneurysm. *Br J Surg.* 2003;90(4):492.

67. Lindholt JS, Juul S, Fasting H, et al. Hospital costs and benefits of screening for abdominal aortic aneurysms. Results from a randomised population screening trial. *Eur J Vasc Endovasc Surg.* 2002;23(1):55-60. PMID: 11748949.

68. Lederle FA, Wilson SE, Johnson GR, et al. Variability in measurement of abdominal aortic aneurysms. Abdominal Aortic Aneurysm Detection and Management Veterans Administration Cooperative Study Group. *J Vasc Surg.* 1995;21(6):945-52. PMID: 7776474.

69. Zarnke MD, Gould HR, Goldman MH. Computed tomography in the evaluation of the patient with symptomatic abdominal aortic aneurysm. *Surgery.* 1988;103(6):638-42. PMID: 3375990.

70. Fink HA, Lederle FA, Roth CS, et al. The accuracy of physical examination to detect abdominal aortic aneurysm. *Arch Intern Med.* 2000;160(6):833-6. PMID: 10737283.

71. Lederle FA, Simel DL. The rational clinical examination. Does this patient have abdominal aortic aneurysm? *JAMA.* 1999;281(1):77-82. PMID: 9892455.

72. Brown LC, Greenhalgh RM, Thompson SG, et al. Does EVAR alter the rate of cardiovascular events in patients with abdominal aortic aneurysm considered unfit for open repair? Results from the randomised EVAR trial 2. *Eur J Vasc Endovasc Surg.* 2010;39(4):396-402. PMID: 20096611.

73. Grootenboer N, Hendriks JM, Cuypers PW, et al. Endovascular abdominal aortic aneurysm repair in women. *Acta Chir Belg.* 2011;111(1):2-6. PMID: 21520779.

74. Parodi JC, Palmaz JC, Barone HD. Transfemoral intraluminal graft implantation for abdominal aortic aneurysms. *Ann Vasc Surg.* 1991;5(6):491-9. PMID: 1837729.

75. Karthikesalingam A, Al-Jundi W, Jackson D, et al. Systematic review and meta-analysis of duplex ultrasonography, contrast-enhanced ultrasonography or computed tomography for surveillance after endovascular aneurysm repair. *Br J Surg.* 2012;99(11):1514-23. PMID: 23001681.

76. Greenhalgh RM, Brown LC, Kwong GP, et al. Comparison of endovascular aneurysm repair with open repair in patients with abdominal aortic aneurysm (EVAR trial 1), 30-day operative mortality results: randomised controlled trial. *Lancet.* 2004;364(9437):843-8. PMID: 15351191.

77. EVAR Trial Participants. Endovascular aneurysm repair versus open repair in patients with abdominal aortic aneurym (EVAR trial 1): randomised controlled trial. *Lancet.* 2005;365(9478):2179-86. PMID: 15978925.

78. United Kingdom EVAR Trial Investigators; Greenhalgh RM, Brown LC, et al. Endovascular versus open repair of abdominal aortic aneurysm. *N Engl J Med.* 2010;362(20):1863-71. PMID: 20382983.

79. Lederle FA, Freischlag JA, Kyriakides TC, et al. Outcomes following endovascular vs open repair of abdominal aortic aneurysm: a randomized trial. *JAMA.* 2009;302(14):1535-42. PMID: 19826022.

80. Prinssen M, Verhoeven EL, Buth J, et al. A randomized trial comparing conventional and endovascular repair of abdominal aortic aneurysms. *N Engl J Med.* 2004;351(16):1607-18. PMID: 15483279.

81. Blankensteijn JD, de Jong SE, Prinssen M, et al. Two-year outcomes after conventional or endovascular repair of abdominal aortic aneurysms. *N Engl J Med.* 2005;352(23):2398-405. PMID: 15944424.

82. EVAR Trial Participants. Endovascular aneurysm repair and outcome in patients unfit for open repair of abdominal aortic aneurysm (EVAR trial 2): randomised controlled trial. *Lancet.* 2005;365(9478):2187-92. PMID: 15978926.

83. United Kingdom EVAR Trial Investigators; Greenhalgh RM, Brown LC, et al. Endovascular repair of aortic aneurysm in patients physically ineligible for open repair. *N Engl J Med.* 2010;362(20):1872-80. PMID: 20382982.

84. Fleming C, Whitlock E, Beil T, et al. Primary Care Screening for Abdominal Aortic Aneurysm. Evidence Synthesis No. 35. Rockville, MD: Agency for Healthcare Research and Quality; 2005. PMID: 20722131.

85. Harris RP, Helfand M, Woolf SH, et al. Current methods of the US Preventive Services Task Force: a review of the process. *Am J Prev Med.* 2001;20(3 Suppl):21-35. PMID: 11306229.

86. U.S. Preventive Services Task Force. U.S. Preventive Services Task Force Procedure Manual. Rockville, MD: Agency for Healthcare Research and Quality; 2013.

87. National Institute for Health and Clinical Excellence. The Guidelines Manual. London: National Institute for Health and Clinical Excellence; 2006.

88. DerSimonian R, Laird N. Meta-analysis in clinical trials. *Control Clin Trials.* 1986;7(3):177-88. PMID: 3802833.

89. Kim LG, P Scott RA, Ashton HA, et al. A sustained mortality benefit from screening for abdominal aortic aneurysm. *Ann Intern Med.* 2007;146(10):699-706. PMID: 17502630.

90. Thompson SG, Ashton HA, Gao L, et al. Screening men for abdominal aortic aneurysm: 10 year mortality and cost effectiveness results from the randomised Multicentre Aneurysm Screening Study. *BMJ.* 2009;338:b2307. PMID: 19553269.

91. Ashton HA, Gao L, Kim LG, et al. Fifteen-year follow-up of a randomized clinical trial of ultrasonographic screening for abdominal aortic aneurysms. *Br J Surg.* 2007;94(6):696-701. PMID: 17514666.

92. Lindholt JS, Juul S, Fasting H, et al. Preliminary ten year results from a randomised single centre mass screening trial for abdominal aortic aneurysm. *Eur J Vasc Endovasc Surg.* 2006;32(6):608-14. PMID: 16893663.

93. Lindholt JS, Sorensen J, Sogaard R, et al. Long-term benefit and cost-effectiveness analysis of screening for abdominal aortic aneurysms from a randomized controlled trial. *Br J Surg.* 2010;97(6):826-34. PMID: 20473995.

94. Lindholt JS, Vammen S, Fasting H, et al. Psychological consequences of screening for abdominal aortic aneurysm and conservative treatment of small abdominal aortic aneurysms. *Eur J Vasc Endovasc Surg.* 2000;20(1):79-83. PMID: 10906303.

95. Spencer CA, Norman PE, Jamrozik K, et al. Is screening for abdominal aortic aneurysm bad for your health and well-being? *ANZ J Surg.* 2004;74(12):1069-75. PMID: 15574151.

96. d'Audiffret A, Santilli S, Tretinyak A, et al. Fate of the ectatic infrarenal aorta: expansion rates and outcomes. *Ann Vasc Surg.* 2002;16(5):534-6. PMID: 12183768.

97. Scott RA, Vardulaki KA, Walker NM, et al. The long-term benefits of a single scan for abdominal aortic aneurysm (AAA) at age 65. *Eur J Vasc Endovasc Surg.* 2001;21(6):535-40. PMID: 11397028.

98. Devaraj S, Dodds SR. Ultrasound surveillance of ectatic abdominal aortas. *Ann R Coll Surg Engl.* 2008;90(6):477-82. PMID: 18765027.

99. Hafez H, Druce PS, Ashton HA. Abdominal aortic aneurysm development in men following a "normal" aortic ultrasound scan. *Eur J Vasc Endovasc Surg.* 2008;36(5):553-8.

PMID: 18718773.

100. Lindholt JS, Vammen S, Juul S, et al. Optimal interval screening and surveillance of abdominal aortic aneurysms. *Eur J Vasc Endovasc Surg.* 2000;20(4):369-73. PMID: 11035969.

101. Lederle FA, Johnson GR, Wilson SE, et al. Yield of repeated screening for abdominal aortic aneurysm after a 4-year interval. Aneurysm Detection and Management Veterans Affairs Cooperative Study Investigators. *Arch Intern Med.* 2000;160(8):1117-21. PMID: 10789604.

102. Emerton ME, Shaw E, Poskitt K, et al. Screening for abdominal aortic aneurysm: a single scan is enough. *Br J Surg.* 1994;81(8):1112-3. PMID: 7953333.

103. Crow P, Shaw E, Earnshaw JJ, et al. A single normal ultrasonographic scan at age 65 years rules out significant aneurysm disease for life in men. *Br J Surg.* 2001;88(7):941-4. PMID: 11442524.

104. Wanhainen A, Rosen C, Rutegard J, et al. Low quality of life prior to screening for abdominal aortic aneurysm: a possible risk factor for negative mental effects. *Ann Vasc Surg.* 2004;18(3):287-93. PMID: 15354629.

105. Lucarotti ME, Heather BP, Shaw E, et al. Psychological morbidity associated with abdominal aortic aneurysm screening. *Eur J Vasc Endovasc Surg.* 1997;14(6):499-501. PMID: 9467527.

106. Lederle FA, Wilson SE, Johnson GR, et al. Immediate repair compared with surveillance of small abdominal aortic aneurysms. *N Engl J Med.* 2002;346(19):1437-44. PMID: 12000813.

107. Lederle FA, Johnson GR, Wilson SE, et al. Quality of life, impotence, and activity level in a randomized trial of immediate repair versus surveillance of small abdominal aortic aneurysm. *J Vasc Surg.* 2003;38(4):745-52. PMID: 14560224.

108. Powell JT, Brady AR, Brown LC, et al. Mortality results for randomised controlled trial of early elective surgery or ultrasonographic surveillance for small abdominal aortic aneurysms. The UK Small Aneurysm Trial Participants. *Lancet.* 1998;352(9141):1649-55. PMID: 9853436.

109. Powell JT, Brown LC, Forbes JF, et al. Final 12-year follow-up of surgery versus surveillance in the UK Small Aneurysm Trial. *Br J Surg.* 2007;94(6):702-8. PMID: 17514693.

110. Brown LC, Thompson SG, Greenhalgh RM, et al. Fit patients with small abdominal aortic aneurysms (AAAs) do not benefit from early intervention. *J Vasc Surg.* 2008;48(6):1375-81. PMID: 19118733.

111. Fowkes FG, Greenhalgh RM, Powell JT, et al. Length of hospital stay following elective abdominal aortic aneurysm repair. U.K. Small Aneurysm Trial Participants. *Eur J Vasc Endovasc Surg.* 1998;16(3):185-91. PMID: 9787298.

112. Sun Z. Diagnostic value of color duplex ultrasonography in the follow-up of endovascular repair of abdominal aortic aneurysm. *J Vasc Interv Radiol.* 2006;17(5):759-64. PMID: 16687740.

113. Cao P, De Rango P, Verzini F, et al. Comparison of surveillance versus aortic endografting for small aneurysm repair (CAESAR): results from a randomised trial. *Eur J Vasc Endovasc Surg.* 2011;41(1):13-25. PMID: 20869890.

114. De Rango P, Verzini F, Parlani G, et al. Quality of life in patients with small abdominal aortic aneurysm: the effect of early endovascular repair versus surveillance in the CAESAR

trial. *Eur J Vasc Endovasc Surg.* 2011;41(3):324-31. PMID: 21145269.

115. Ouriel K, Clair DG, Kent KC, et al. Endovascular repair compared with surveillance for patients with small abdominal aortic aneurysms. *J Vasc Surg.* 2010;51(5):1081-7. PMID: 20304589.

116. Propanolol Aneurysm Trial Investigators. Propranolol for small abdominal aortic aneurysms: results of a randomized trial. *J Vasc Surg.* 2002;35(1):72-9. PMID: 11802135.

117. Lindholt JS, Henneberg EW, Juul S, et al. Impaired results of a randomised double blinded clinical trial of propranolol versus placebo on the expansion rate of small abdominal aortic aneurysms. *Int Angiol.* 1999;18(1):52-7. PMID: 10392481.

118. Mosorin M, Juvonen J, Biancari F, et al. Use of doxycycline to decrease the growth rate of abdominal aortic aneurysms: a randomized, double-blind, placebo-controlled pilot study. *J Vasc Surg.* 2001;34(4):606-10. PMID: 11668312.

119. Karlsson L, Gnarpe J, Bergqvist D, et al. The effect of azithromycin and Chlamydophilia pneumonia infection on expansion of small abdominal aortic aneurysms—a prospective randomized double-blind trial. *J Vasc Surg.* 2009;50(1):23-9. PMID: 19563951.

120. Vammen S, Lindholt JS, Ostergaard L, et al. Randomized double-blind controlled trial of roxithromycin for prevention of abdominal aortic aneurysm expansion. *Br J Surg.* 2001;88(8):1066-72. PMID: 11488791.

121. Hogh A, Vammen S, Ostergaard L, et al. Intermittent roxithromycin for preventing progression of small abdominal aortic aneurysms: long-term results of a small clinical trial. *Vasc Endovascular Surg.* 2009;43(5):452-6. PMID: 19640922.

122. Golledge J, Parr A, Boult M, et al. The outcome of endovascular repair of small abdominal aortic aneurysms. *Ann Surg.* 2007;245(2):326-33. PMID: 17245188.

123. Peppelenbosch N, Buth J, Harris PL, et al. Diameter of abdominal aortic aneurysm and outcome of endovascular aneurysm repair: does size matter? A report from EUROSTAR. *J Vasc Surg.* 2004;39(2):288-97. PMID: 14743127.

124. Vardulaki KA, Walker NM, Couto E, et al. Late results concerning feasibility and compliance from a randomized trial of ultrasonographic screening for abdominal aortic aneurysm. *Br J Surg.* 2002;89(7):861-4. PMID: 12081734.

125. Lindholt JS, Juul S, Henneberg EW. High-risk and low-risk screening for abdominal aortic aneurysm both reduce aneurysm-related mortality. A stratified analysis from a single-centre randomised screening trial. *Eur J Vasc Endovasc Surg.* 2007;34(1):53-8. PMID: 17331750.

126. McCarthy RJ, Shaw E, Whyman MR, et al. Recommendations for screening intervals for small aortic aneurysms. *Br J Surg.* 2003;90(7):821-6. PMID: 12854107.

127. Wild JB, Stather PW, Biancari F, et al. A multicentre observational study of the outcomes of screening detected sub-aneurysmal aortic dilatation. *Eur J Vasc Endovasc Surg.* 2013;45(2):128-34. PMID: 23273900.

128. Lesjak M, Boreland F, Lyle D, et al. Screening for abdominal aortic aneurysm: does it affect men's quality of life? *Aust J Prim Health.* 2012;18(4):284-8. PMID: 22951209.

129. Thompson SG, Ashton HA, Gao L, et al. Final follow-up of the Multicentre Aneurysm Screening Study (MASS) randomized trial of abdominal aortic aneurysm screening. *Br J Surg.* 2012;99(12):1649-56. PMID: 23034729.

130. Hassen TA, Pearson S, Cowled PA, et al. Preoperative nutritional status predicts the severity of the systemic inflammatory response syndrome (SIRS) following major vascular surgery. *Eur J Vasc Endovasc Surg.* 2007;33(6):696-702. PMID: 17276097.

131. Yusuf S, Wittes J, Probstfield J, et al. Analysis and interpretation of treatment effects in

subgroups of patients in randomized clinical trials. *JAMA.* 1991;266(1):93-8. PMID: 2046134.

132. Forbes JF, Brady AR, Brown LC, et al. Health service costs and quality of life for early elective surgery or ultrasonographic surveillance for small abdominal aortic aneurysms. UK Small Aneurysm Trial Participants. *Lancet.* 1998;352(9141):1656-60. PMID: 9853437.

133. Stewart AL, Greenfield S, Hays RD, et al. Functional status and well-being of patients with chronic conditions. Results from the Medical Outcomes Study. *JAMA.* 1989;262(7):907-13. PMID: 2754790.

134. Lindholt JS, Norman P. Screening for abdominal aortic aneurysm reduces overall mortality in men. A meta-analysis of the mid- and long-term effects of screening for abdominal aortic aneurysms. *Eur J Vasc Endovasc Surg.* 2008;36(2):167-71. PMID: 18485756.

135. Takagi H, Goto SN, Matsui M, et al. A further meta-analysis of population-based screening for abdominal aortic aneurysm. *J Vasc Surg.* 2010;52(4):1103-8. PMID: 20541347.

136. Cosford PA, Leng GC. Screening for abdominal aortic aneurysm. *Cochrane Database Syst Rev.* 2007;(2):CD002945. PMID: 17443519.

137. Lederle FA. Comment on "Screening for abdominal aortic aneurysm reduces overall mortality in men." *Eur J Vasc Endovasc Surg.* 2008;36(5):620-1. PMID: 18774311.

138. Takagi H, Niwa M, Mizuno Y, et al. The last judgment upon abdominal aortic aneurysm screening. *Int J Cardiol.* 2013;167(5):2331-2. PMID: 23174171.

139. McPhee JT, Hill JS, Eslami MH. The impact of gender on presentation, therapy, and mortality of abdominal aortic aneurysm in the United States, 2001–2004. *J Vasc Surg.* 2007;45(5):891-9. PMID: 17391899.

140. Heikkinen M, Salenius JP, Auvinen O. Ruptured abdominal aortic aneurysm in a well-defined geographic area. *J Vasc Surg.* 2002;36(2):291-6. PMID: 12170209.

141. Forbes TL, Lawlor DK, DeRose G, et al. Gender differences in relative dilatation of abdominal aortic aneurysms. *Ann Vasc Surg.* 2006;20(5):564-8. PMID: 16741651.

142. Acosta S, Ogren M, Bengtsson H, et al. Increasing incidence of ruptured abdominal aortic aneurysm: a population-based study. *J Vasc Surg.* 2006;44(2):237-43. PMID: 16890847.

143. Sandgren T, Sonesson B, Ahlgren R, et al. The diameter of the common femoral artery in healthy human: influence of sex, age, and body size. *J Vasc Surg.* 1999;29(3):503-10. PMID: 10069915.

144. Lederle FA, Johnson GR, Wilson SE, et al. Prevalence and associations of abdominal aortic aneurysm detected through screening. Aneurysm Detection and Management (ADAM) Veterans Affairs Cooperative Study Group. *Ann Intern Med.* 1997;126(6):441-9. PMID: 9072929.

145. Pirie K, Peto R, Reeves GK, et al. The 21st century hazards of smoking and benefits of stopping: a prospective study of one million women in the UK. *Lancet.* 2013;381(9861):133-41. PMID: 23107252.

146. Svensjo S, Bjorck M, Wanhainen A. Current prevalence of abdominal aortic aneurysm in 70-year-old women. *Br J Surg.* 2013;100(3):367-72. PMID: 23192439.

147. Linne A, Lindstrom D, Hultgren R. High prevalence of abdominal aortic aneurysms in brothers and sisters of patients despite a low prevalence in the population. *J Vasc Surg.* 2012;56(2):305-10.

148. Ogata T, MacKean GL, Cole CW, et al. The lifetime prevalence of abdominal aortic aneurysms among siblings of aneurysm patients is eightfold higher than among siblings of spouses: an analysis of 187 aneurysm families in Nova Scotia, Canada. *J Vasc Surg.*

2005;42(5):891-7. PMID: 16275443.

149. Badger SA, O'Donnell ME, Boyd CS, et al. The low prevalence of abdominal aortic aneurysm in relatives in Northern Ireland. *Eur J Vasc Endovasc Surg.* 2007;34(2):163-8. PMID: 17470405.

150. Mureebe L, Egorova N, Giacovelli JK, et al. National trends in the repair of ruptured abdominal aortic aneurysms. *J Vasc Surg.* 2008;48(5):1101-7. PMID: 18771883.

151. Kung HC, Hoyert DL, Xu J, et al. Deaths: final data for 2005. *Natl Vital Stat Rep.* 2008;56(10):1-120. PMID: 18512336.

152. Longo C, Upchurch GR Jr. Abdominal aortic aneurysm screening: recommendations and controversies. *Vasc Endovascular Surg.* 2005;39(3):213-9. PMID: 15920649.

153. Hanly AM, Javad S, Anderson LP, et al. Screening for abdominal aortic aneurysms in cardiovascular patients. *J Surg Res.* 2006;132(1):52-5. PMID: 16171823.

154. Badger SA, O'Donnell ME, Sharif MA, et al. Advantages and pitfalls of abdominal aortic aneurysm screening in high-risk patients. *Vascular.* 2008;16(421):201-6. PMID: 18845100.

155. Mani K, Alund M, Bjorck M, et al. Screening for abdominal aortic aneurysm among patients referred to the vascular laboratory is cost-effective. *Eur J Vasc Endovasc Surg.* 2010;39(2):208-16. PMID: 19942460.

156. Spencer CA, Jamrozik K, Norman PE, et al. The potential for a selective screening strategy for abdominal aortic aneurysm. *J Med Screen.* 2000;7(4):209-11. PMID: 11202589.

157. Kent KC, Zwolak RM, Egorova NN, et al. Analysis of risk factors for abdominal aortic aneurysm in a cohort of more than 3 million individuals. *J Vasc Surg.* 2010;52(3):539-48. PMID: 20630687.

158. Greco G, Egorova NN, Gelijns AC, et al. Development of a novel scoring tool for the identification of large ≥5 cm abdominal aortic aneurysms. *Ann Surg.* 2010;252(4):675-82. PMID: 20881774.

159. Mell M, White JJ, Hill BB, et al. No increased mortality with early aortic aneurysm disease. *J Vasc Surg.* 2012;56(5):1246-51. PMID: 22832264.

160. Robbins DA. Current modalities for abdominal aortic aneurysm repair: implications for nurses. *J Vasc Nurs.* 2010;28(4):136-46. PMID: 21074116.

161. Altman DG, Vergouwe Y, Royston P, et al. Prognosis and prognostic research: validating a prognostic model. *BMJ.* 2009;338:b605. PMID: 19477892.

162. Cook NR. Assessing the incremental role of novel and emerging risk factors. *Curr Cardiovasc Risk Rep.* 2010;4(2):112-9. PMID: 20640227.

163. Mell MW, Hlatky MA, Shreibati JB, et al. Late diagnosis of abdominal aortic aneurysms substantiates underutilization of abdominal aortic aneurysm screening for Medicare beneficiaries. *J Vasc Surg.* 2013;57(6):1519-23. PMID: 23414696.

164. Lederle FA. The rise and fall of abdominal aortic aneurysm. *Circulation.* 2011;124(10):1097-9. PMID: 21900095.

165. Anjum A, von Allmen R, Greenhalgh R, et al. Explaining the decrease in mortality from abdominal aortic aneurysm rupture. *Br J Surg.* 2012;99(5):637-45. PMID: 22473277.

166. Chun KC, Teng KY, Van Spyk EN, et al. Outcomes of an abdominal aortic aneurysm screening program. *J Vac Surg.* 2013;57(2):376-81. PMID: 23141680.

167. Mastracci TM, Cina CS. Screening for abdominal aortic aneurysm in Canada: review and position statement of the Canadian Society for Vascular Surgery. *J Vasc Surg.* 2007;45(6):1268-76. PMID: 17543696.

168. Hirsch AT, Haskal ZJ, Hertzer NR, et al. ACC/AHA 2005 practice guidelines for the

management of patients with peripheral arterial disease (lower extremity, renal, mesenteric, and abdominal aortic). *Circulation.* 2005;113:e463-654.

169. Abramson BL, Hucknell V, Anand S, et al. 2005 Canadian Cardiovascular Society Consensus Conference: peripheral arterial disease—executive summary. *Can J Cardiol.* 2005;21:997-1006.

170. Ballard DJ, Filardo G, Fowkes G, et al. Surgery for small asymptomatic abdominal aortic aneurysms. *Cochrane Database Syst Rev.* 2008(4):CD001835. PMID: 18843626.

171. Rughani G, Robertson L, Clarke M. Medical treatment for small abdominal aortic aneurysms. *Cochrane Database Syst Rev.* 2012;(9):CD009536.

172. Hassan C, Pickhardt PJ, Laghi A, et al. Computed tomographic colonography to screen for colorectal cancer, extracolonic cancer, and aortic aneurysm: model simulation with cost-effectiveness analysis. *Arch Intern Med.* 2008;168(7):696-705. PMID: 18413551.

173. Xiong T, Richardson M, Woodroffe R, et al. Incidental lesions found on CT colonography: their nature and frequency. *Br J Radiol.* 2005;78(925):22-9. PMID: 15673525.

174. van Walraven C, Wong J, Morant K, et al. The influence of incidental abdominal aortic aneurysm monitoring on patient outcomes. *J Vasc Surg.* 2011;54(5):1290-7. PMID: 21803526.

175. Gordon JR, Wahls T, Carlos RC, et al. Failure to recognize newly identified aortic dilations in a health care system with an advanced electronic medical record. *Ann Intern Med.* 2009;151(1):21-7. PMID: 19581643.

176. Forsdahl SH, Solberg S, Singh K, et al. Abdominal aortic aneurysms, or a relatively large diameter of non-aneurysmal aortas, increase total and cardiovascular mortality: the Tromso study. *Int J Epidemiol.* 2010;39(1):225-32. PMID: 19897467.

177. Freiberg MS, Arnold AM, Newman AB, et al. Abdominal aortic aneurysms, increasing infrarenal aortic diameter, and risk of total mortality and incident cardiovascular disease events: 10-year follow-up data from the Cardiovascular Health Study. *Circulation.* 2008;117(8):1010-7. PMID: 18268154.

178. Grondal N, Sogaard R, Henneberg EW, et al. The Viborg Vascular (VIVA) screening trial of 65–74 year old men in the central region of Denmark: study protocol. *Trials.* 2010;11:67. PMID: 20507582.

179. Twine CP, Williams IM. Systematic review and meta-analysis of the effects of statin therapy on abdominal aortic aneurysms. *Br J Surg.* 2011;98(3):346-53. PMID: 21254006.

Figure 1. Analytic Framework

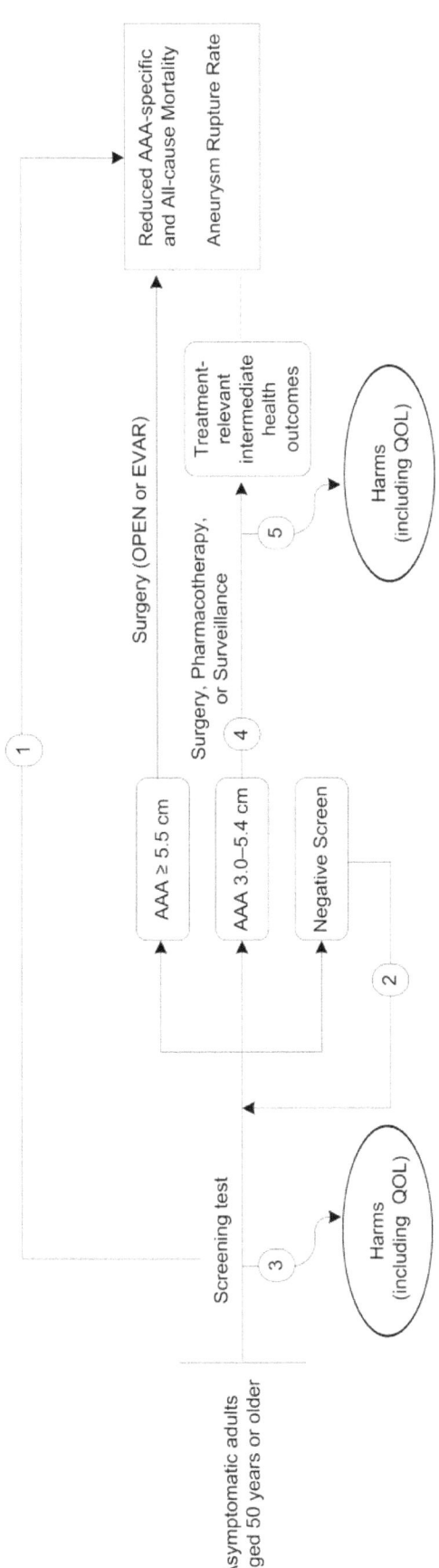

Abbreviations: AAA = abdominal aortic aneurysm; EVAR = endovascular aneurysm repair; OPEN = open abdominal aortic aneurysm repair; QOL = quality of life.

Figure 2. Pooled Analysis of AAA-Related Mortality in One-Time Screening Trials (Random-Effects Model)

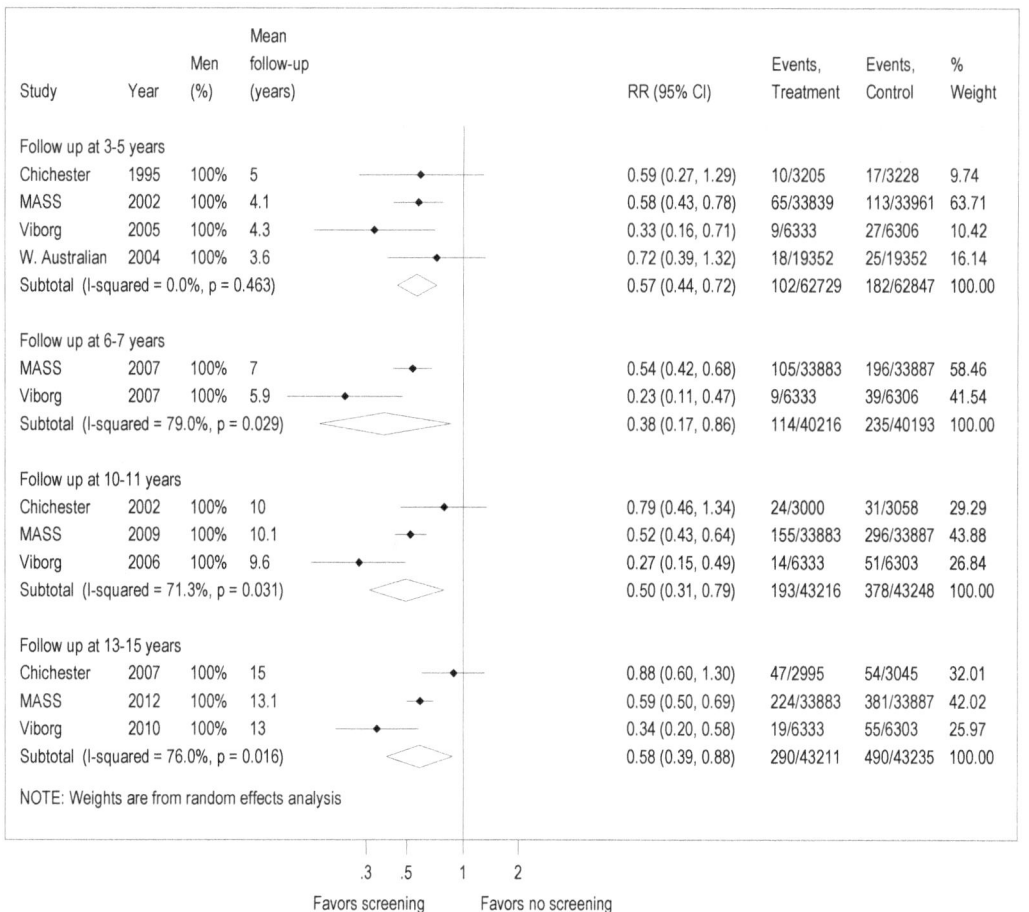

Study	Year	Men (%)	Mean follow-up (years)	RR (95% CI)	Events, Treatment	Events, Control	% Weight
Follow up at 3-5 years							
Chichester	1995	100%	5	0.59 (0.27, 1.29)	10/3205	17/3228	9.74
MASS	2002	100%	4.1	0.58 (0.43, 0.78)	65/33839	113/33961	63.71
Viborg	2005	100%	4.3	0.33 (0.16, 0.71)	9/6333	27/6306	10.42
W. Australian	2004	100%	3.6	0.72 (0.39, 1.32)	18/19352	25/19352	16.14
Subtotal (I-squared = 0.0%, p = 0.463)				0.57 (0.44, 0.72)	102/62729	182/62847	100.00
Follow up at 6-7 years							
MASS	2007	100%	7	0.54 (0.42, 0.68)	105/33883	196/33887	58.46
Viborg	2007	100%	5.9	0.23 (0.11, 0.47)	9/6333	39/6306	41.54
Subtotal (I-squared = 79.0%, p = 0.029)				0.38 (0.17, 0.86)	114/40216	235/40193	100.00
Follow up at 10-11 years							
Chichester	2002	100%	10	0.79 (0.46, 1.34)	24/3000	31/3058	29.29
MASS	2009	100%	10.1	0.52 (0.43, 0.64)	155/33883	296/33887	43.88
Viborg	2006	100%	9.6	0.27 (0.15, 0.49)	14/6333	51/6303	26.84
Subtotal (I-squared = 71.3%, p = 0.031)				0.50 (0.31, 0.79)	193/43216	378/43248	100.00
Follow up at 13-15 years							
Chichester	2007	100%	15	0.88 (0.60, 1.30)	47/2995	54/3045	32.01
MASS	2012	100%	13.1	0.59 (0.50, 0.69)	224/33883	381/33887	42.02
Viborg	2010	100%	13	0.34 (0.20, 0.58)	19/6333	55/6303	25.97
Subtotal (I-squared = 76.0%, p = 0.016)				0.58 (0.39, 0.88)	290/43211	490/43235	100.00

NOTE: Weights are from random effects analysis

.3   .5   1   2

Favors screening   Favors no screening

Figure 3. Pooled Analysis of All-Cause Mortality in Screening Trials (Random-Effects Model)

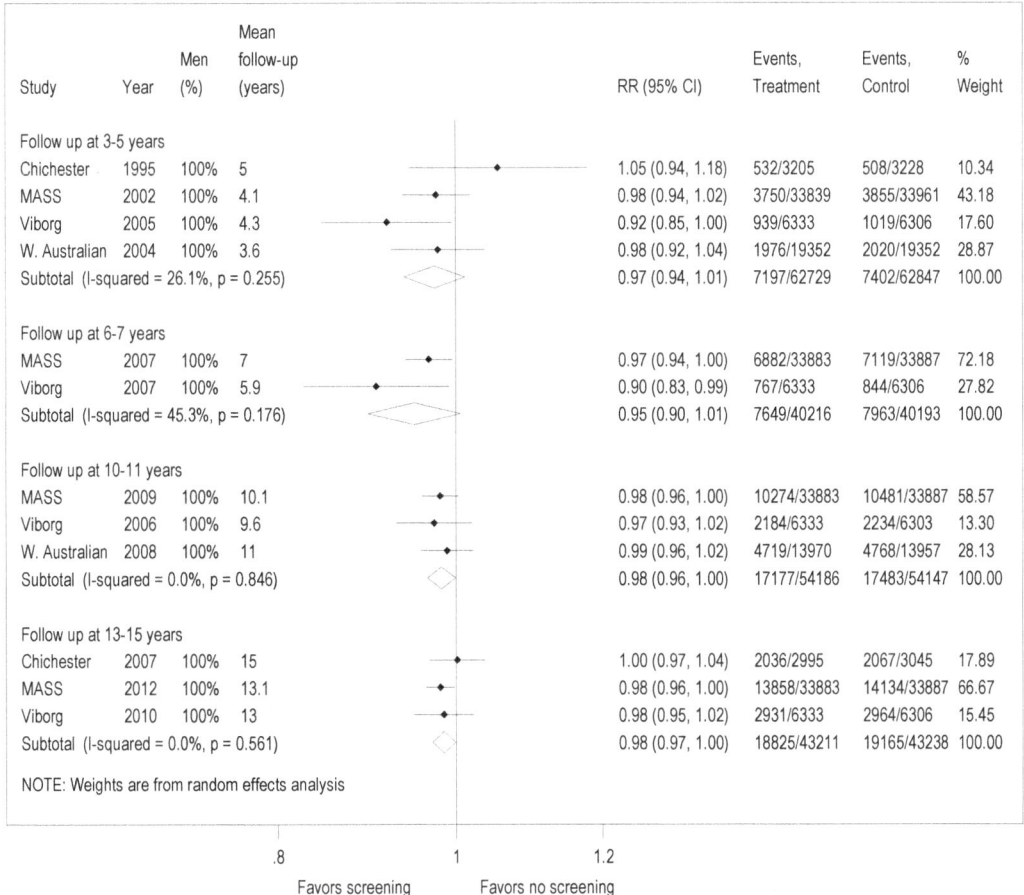

Study	Year	Men (%)	Mean follow-up (years)	RR (95% CI)	Events, Treatment	Events, Control	% Weight
Follow up at 3-5 years							
Chichester	1995	100%	5	1.05 (0.94, 1.18)	532/3205	508/3228	10.34
MASS	2002	100%	4.1	0.98 (0.94, 1.02)	3750/33839	3855/33961	43.18
Viborg	2005	100%	4.3	0.92 (0.85, 1.00)	939/6333	1019/6306	17.60
W. Australian	2004	100%	3.6	0.98 (0.92, 1.04)	1976/19352	2020/19352	28.87
Subtotal (I-squared = 26.1%, p = 0.255)				0.97 (0.94, 1.01)	7197/62729	7402/62847	100.00
Follow up at 6-7 years							
MASS	2007	100%	7	0.97 (0.94, 1.00)	6882/33883	7119/33887	72.18
Viborg	2007	100%	5.9	0.90 (0.83, 0.99)	767/6333	844/6306	27.82
Subtotal (I-squared = 45.3%, p = 0.176)				0.95 (0.90, 1.01)	7649/40216	7963/40193	100.00
Follow up at 10-11 years							
MASS	2009	100%	10.1	0.98 (0.96, 1.00)	10274/33883	10481/33887	58.57
Viborg	2006	100%	9.6	0.97 (0.93, 1.02)	2184/6333	2234/6303	13.30
W. Australian	2008	100%	11	0.99 (0.96, 1.02)	4719/13970	4768/13957	28.13
Subtotal (I-squared = 0.0%, p = 0.846)				0.98 (0.96, 1.00)	17177/54186	17483/54147	100.00
Follow up at 13-15 years							
Chichester	2007	100%	15	1.00 (0.97, 1.04)	2036/2995	2067/3045	17.89
MASS	2012	100%	13.1	0.98 (0.96, 1.00)	13858/33883	14134/33887	66.67
Viborg	2010	100%	13	0.98 (0.95, 1.02)	2931/6333	2964/6306	15.45
Subtotal (I-squared = 0.0%, p = 0.561)				0.98 (0.97, 1.00)	18825/43211	19165/43238	100.00

NOTE: Weights are from random effects analysis

.8   1   1.2

Favors screening   Favors no screening

Figure 4. Pooled Analysis of Rupture in One-Time Screening Trials (Random-Effects Model)

Study	Year	Men (%)	Mean follow-up (years)		RR (95% CI)	Events, Treatment	Events, Control	% Weight
Follow up at 3-5 years								
Chichester	1995	100%	5		0.45 (0.21, 0.99)	9/3205	20/3228	17.14
MASS	2002	100%	4.1		0.51 (0.38, 0.69)	67/33839	131/33961	36.89
Viborg	2005	100%	4.3		0.27 (0.13, 0.60)	8/6333	29/6306	17.23
W. Australian	2004	100%	3.6		0.87 (0.54, 1.38)	33/19352	38/19352	28.73
Subtotal (I-squared = 58.2%, p = 0.066)					0.52 (0.35, 0.79)	117/62729	218/62847	100.00
Follow up at 6-7 years								
MASS	2007	100%	7		0.53 (0.43, 0.65)	135/33883	257/33887	100.00
Subtotal (I-squared = .%, p = .)					0.53 (0.43, 0.65)	135/33883	257/33887	100.00
Follow up at 10-11 years								
Chichester	2002	100%	10		0.10 (0.03, 0.32)	3/3000	31/3058	24.10
MASS	2009	100%	10.1		0.53 (0.44, 0.63)	197/33883	374/33887	41.59
Viborg	2006	100%	9.6		0.24 (0.12, 0.46)	11/6333	46/6306	34.30
Subtotal (I-squared = 84.0%, p = 0.002)					0.27 (0.11, 0.65)	211/43216	451/43251	100.00
Follow up at 13-15 years								
Chichester	2007	100%	15		0.87 (0.61, 1.25)	54/2995	63/3045	41.99
MASS	2012	100%	13.1		0.57 (0.49, 0.67)	273/33883	476/33887	58.01
Subtotal (I-squared = 77.5%, p = 0.035)					0.68 (0.46, 1.02)	327/36878	539/36932	100.00

NOTE: Weights are from random effects analysis

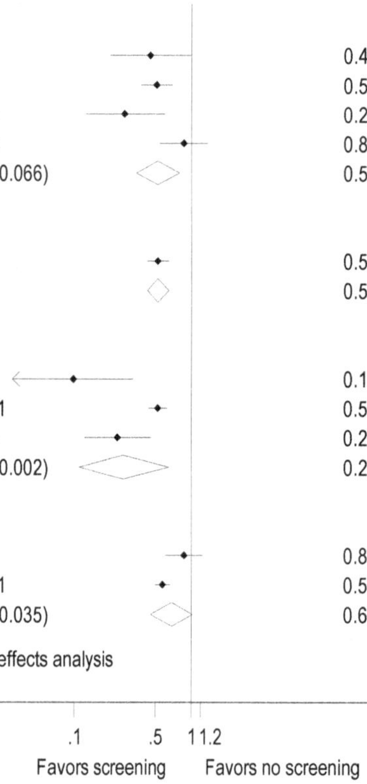

.1   .5   11.2

Favors screening   Favors no screening

Figure 5. Pooled Analysis of Emergent Repairs for Ruptures in One-Time Screening Trials (Random-Effects Model)

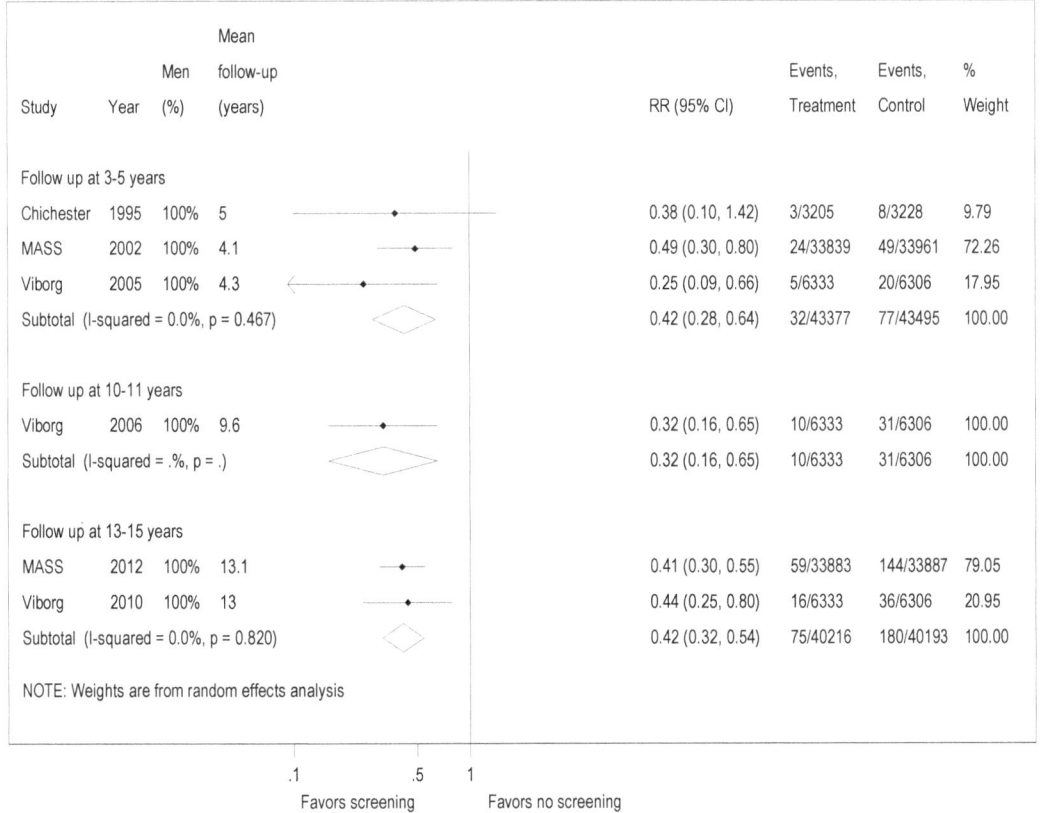

Study	Year	Men (%)	Mean follow-up (years)	RR (95% CI)	Events, Treatment	Events, Control	% Weight
Follow up at 3-5 years							
Chichester	1995	100%	5	0.38 (0.10, 1.42)	3/3205	8/3228	9.79
MASS	2002	100%	4.1	0.49 (0.30, 0.80)	24/33839	49/33961	72.26
Viborg	2005	100%	4.3	0.25 (0.09, 0.66)	5/6333	20/6306	17.95
Subtotal (I-squared = 0.0%, p = 0.467)				0.42 (0.28, 0.64)	32/43377	77/43495	100.00
Follow up at 10-11 years							
Viborg	2006	100%	9.6	0.32 (0.16, 0.65)	10/6333	31/6306	100.00
Subtotal (I-squared = .%, p = .)				0.32 (0.16, 0.65)	10/6333	31/6306	100.00
Follow up at 13-15 years							
MASS	2012	100%	13.1	0.41 (0.30, 0.55)	59/33883	144/33887	79.05
Viborg	2010	100%	13	0.44 (0.25, 0.80)	16/6333	36/6306	20.95
Subtotal (I-squared = 0.0%, p = 0.820)				0.42 (0.32, 0.54)	75/40216	180/40193	100.00

NOTE: Weights are from random effects analysis

.1   .5   1

Favors screening   Favors no screening

Figure 6. Pooled Analysis of 30-Day Mortality in One-Time Screening Trials (Random-Effects Model)

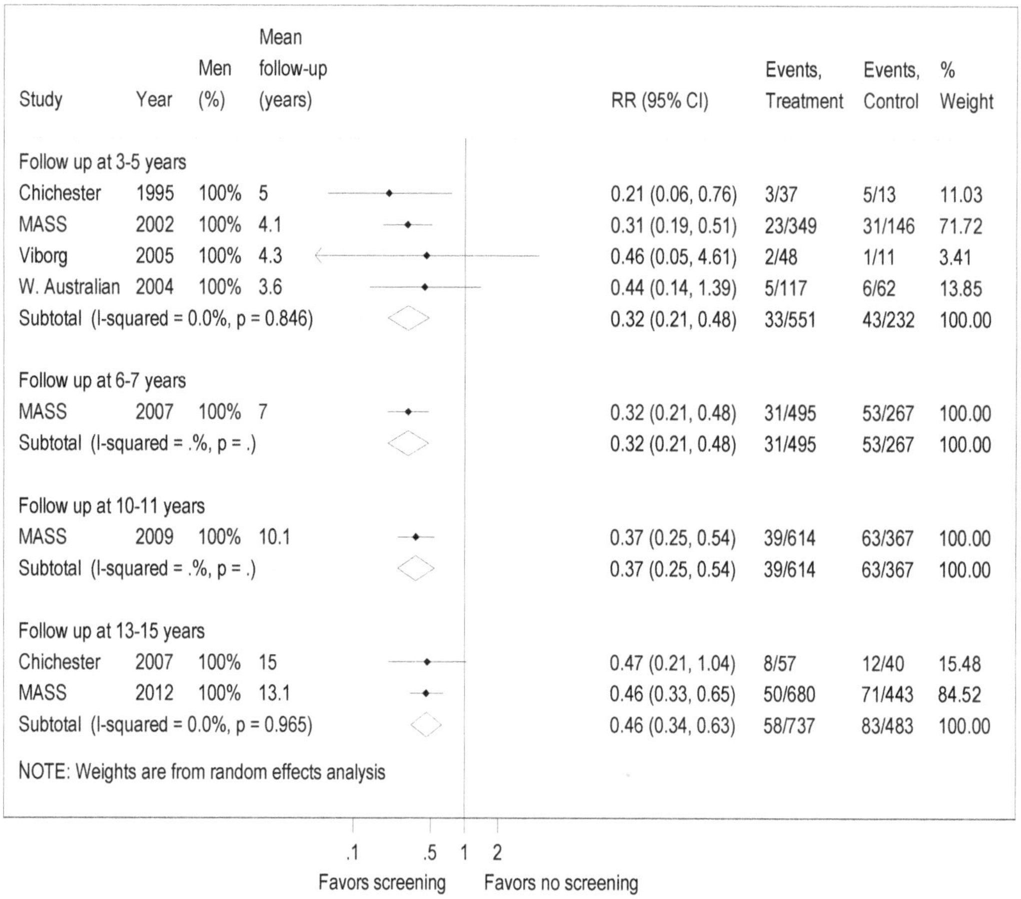

Study	Year	Men (%)	Mean follow-up (years)		RR (95% CI)	Events, Treatment	Events, Control	% Weight
Follow up at 3-5 years								
Chichester	1995	100%	5		0.21 (0.06, 0.76)	3/37	5/13	11.03
MASS	2002	100%	4.1		0.31 (0.19, 0.51)	23/349	31/146	71.72
Viborg	2005	100%	4.3		0.46 (0.05, 4.61)	2/48	1/11	3.41
W. Australian	2004	100%	3.6		0.44 (0.14, 1.39)	5/117	6/62	13.85
Subtotal (I-squared = 0.0%, p = 0.846)					0.32 (0.21, 0.48)	33/551	43/232	100.00
Follow up at 6-7 years								
MASS	2007	100%	7		0.32 (0.21, 0.48)	31/495	53/267	100.00
Subtotal (I-squared = .%, p = .)					0.32 (0.21, 0.48)	31/495	53/267	100.00
Follow up at 10-11 years								
MASS	2009	100%	10.1		0.37 (0.25, 0.54)	39/614	63/367	100.00
Subtotal (I-squared = .%, p = .)					0.37 (0.25, 0.54)	39/614	63/367	100.00
Follow up at 13-15 years								
Chichester	2007	100%	15		0.47 (0.21, 1.04)	8/57	12/40	15.48
MASS	2012	100%	13.1		0.46 (0.33, 0.65)	50/680	71/443	84.52
Subtotal (I-squared = 0.0%, p = 0.965)					0.46 (0.34, 0.63)	58/737	83/483	100.00

NOTE: Weights are from random effects analysis

.1　.5　1　2

Favors screening　　Favors no screening

Figure 7. Pooled Analysis of 30-Day Mortality Due to Elective Surgery in One-Time Screening Trials (Random-Effects Model)

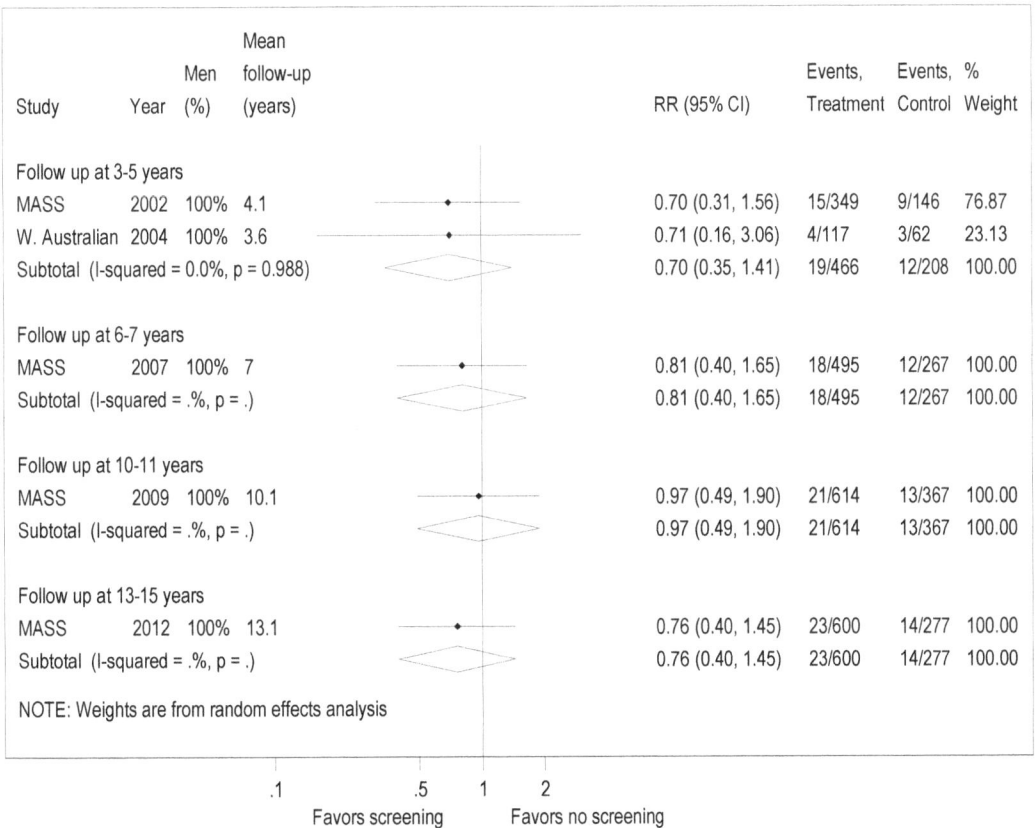

NOTE: Weights are from random effects analysis

Figure 8. Pooled Analysis of 30-Day Mortality Due to Emergency Surgery in One-Time Screening Trials (Random-Effects Model)

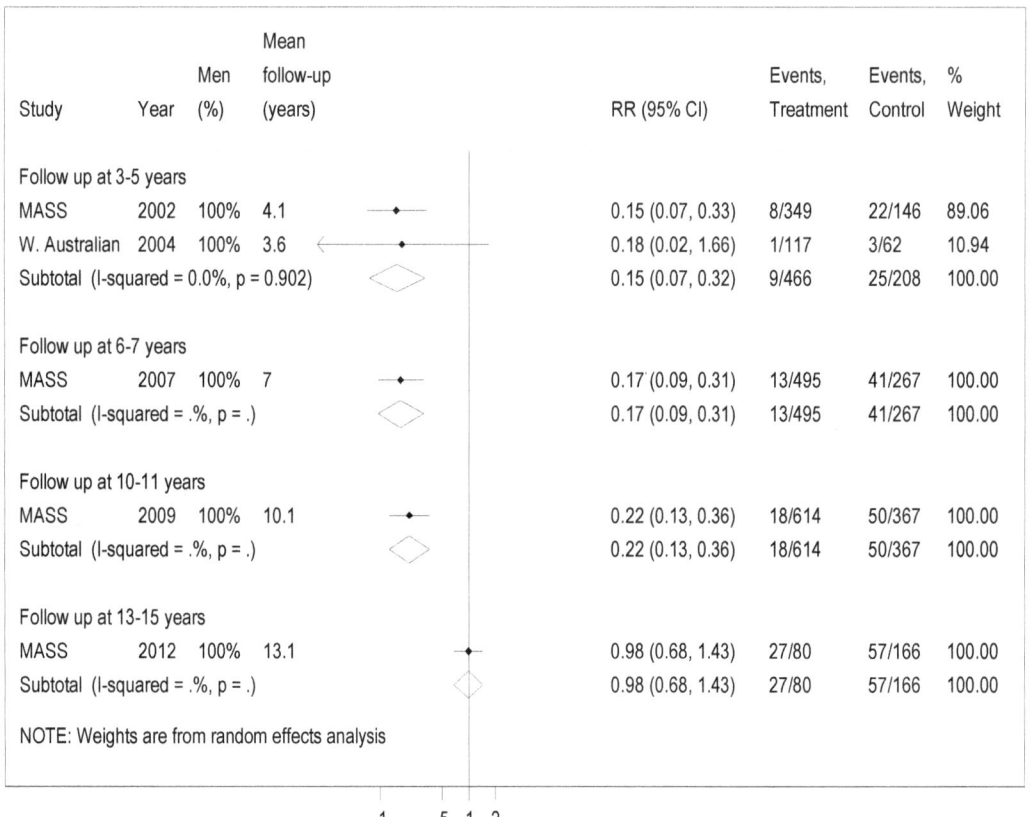

Study	Year	Men (%)	Mean follow-up (years)	RR (95% CI)	Events, Treatment	Events, Control	% Weight
Follow up at 3-5 years							
MASS	2002	100%	4.1	0.15 (0.07, 0.33)	8/349	22/146	89.06
W. Australian	2004	100%	3.6	0.18 (0.02, 1.66)	1/117	3/62	10.94
Subtotal (I-squared = 0.0%, p = 0.902)				0.15 (0.07, 0.32)	9/466	25/208	100.00
Follow up at 6-7 years							
MASS	2007	100%	7	0.17 (0.09, 0.31)	13/495	41/267	100.00
Subtotal (I-squared = .%, p = .)				0.17 (0.09, 0.31)	13/495	41/267	100.00
Follow up at 10-11 years							
MASS	2009	100%	10.1	0.22 (0.13, 0.36)	18/614	50/367	100.00
Subtotal (I-squared = .%, p = .)				0.22 (0.13, 0.36)	18/614	50/367	100.00
Follow up at 13-15 years							
MASS	2012	100%	13.1	0.98 (0.68, 1.43)	27/80	57/166	100.00
Subtotal (I-squared = .%, p = .)				0.98 (0.68, 1.43)	27/80	57/166	100.00

NOTE: Weights are from random effects analysis

.1   .5   1   2

Favors screening   Favors no screening

Figure 9. Pooled Analysis of AAA Operations in One-Time Screening Trials (Random-Effects Model)

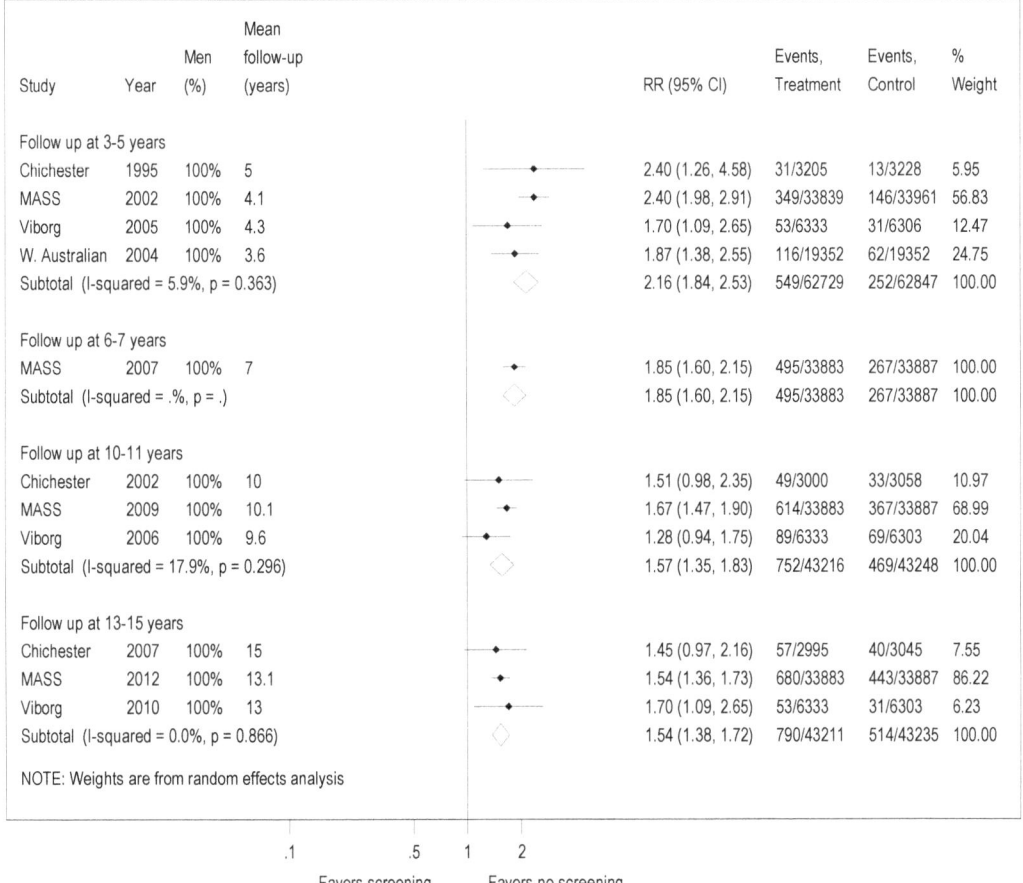

Study	Year	Men (%)	Mean follow-up (years)	RR (95% CI)	Events, Treatment	Events, Control	% Weight
Follow up at 3-5 years							
Chichester	1995	100%	5	2.40 (1.26, 4.58)	31/3205	13/3228	5.95
MASS	2002	100%	4.1	2.40 (1.98, 2.91)	349/33839	146/33961	56.83
Viborg	2005	100%	4.3	1.70 (1.09, 2.65)	53/6333	31/6306	12.47
W. Australian	2004	100%	3.6	1.87 (1.38, 2.55)	116/19352	62/19352	24.75
Subtotal (I-squared = 5.9%, p = 0.363)				2.16 (1.84, 2.53)	549/62729	252/62847	100.00
Follow up at 6-7 years							
MASS	2007	100%	7	1.85 (1.60, 2.15)	495/33883	267/33887	100.00
Subtotal (I-squared = .%, p = .)				1.85 (1.60, 2.15)	495/33883	267/33887	100.00
Follow up at 10-11 years							
Chichester	2002	100%	10	1.51 (0.98, 2.35)	49/3000	33/3058	10.97
MASS	2009	100%	10.1	1.67 (1.47, 1.90)	614/33883	367/33887	68.99
Viborg	2006	100%	9.6	1.28 (0.94, 1.75)	89/6333	69/6303	20.04
Subtotal (I-squared = 17.9%, p = 0.296)				1.57 (1.35, 1.83)	752/43216	469/43248	100.00
Follow up at 13-15 years							
Chichester	2007	100%	15	1.45 (0.97, 2.16)	57/2995	40/3045	7.55
MASS	2012	100%	13.1	1.54 (1.36, 1.73)	680/33883	443/33887	86.22
Viborg	2010	100%	13	1.70 (1.09, 2.65)	53/6333	31/6303	6.23
Subtotal (I-squared = 0.0%, p = 0.866)				1.54 (1.38, 1.72)	790/43211	514/43235	100.00

NOTE: Weights are from random effects analysis

.1   .5   1   2

Favors screening   Favors no screening

Figure 10. Pooled Analysis of Elective Operations in One-Time Screening Trials (Random-Effects Model)

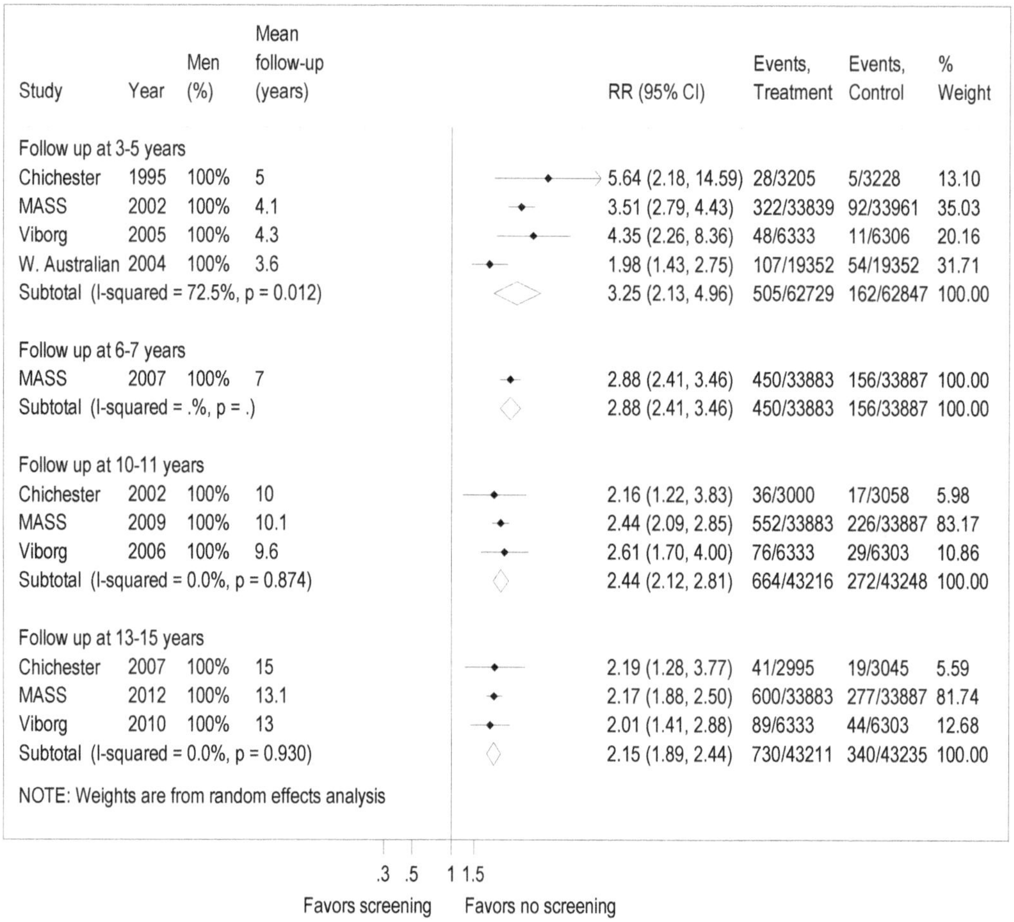

Study	Year	Men (%)	Mean follow-up (years)	RR (95% CI)	Events, Treatment	Events, Control	% Weight
Follow up at 3-5 years							
Chichester	1995	100%	5	5.64 (2.18, 14.59)	28/3205	5/3228	13.10
MASS	2002	100%	4.1	3.51 (2.79, 4.43)	322/33839	92/33961	35.03
Viborg	2005	100%	4.3	4.35 (2.26, 8.36)	48/6333	11/6306	20.16
W. Australian	2004	100%	3.6	1.98 (1.43, 2.75)	107/19352	54/19352	31.71
Subtotal (I-squared = 72.5%, p = 0.012)				3.25 (2.13, 4.96)	505/62729	162/62847	100.00
Follow up at 6-7 years							
MASS	2007	100%	7	2.88 (2.41, 3.46)	450/33883	156/33887	100.00
Subtotal (I-squared = .%, p = .)				2.88 (2.41, 3.46)	450/33883	156/33887	100.00
Follow up at 10-11 years							
Chichester	2002	100%	10	2.16 (1.22, 3.83)	36/3000	17/3058	5.98
MASS	2009	100%	10.1	2.44 (2.09, 2.85)	552/33883	226/33887	83.17
Viborg	2006	100%	9.6	2.61 (1.70, 4.00)	76/6333	29/6303	10.86
Subtotal (I-squared = 0.0%, p = 0.874)				2.44 (2.12, 2.81)	664/43216	272/43248	100.00
Follow up at 13-15 years							
Chichester	2007	100%	15	2.19 (1.28, 3.77)	41/2995	19/3045	5.59
MASS	2012	100%	13.1	2.17 (1.88, 2.50)	600/33883	277/33887	81.74
Viborg	2010	100%	13	2.01 (1.41, 2.88)	89/6333	44/6303	12.68
Subtotal (I-squared = 0.0%, p = 0.930)				2.15 (1.89, 2.44)	730/43211	340/43235	100.00

NOTE: Weights are from random effects analysis

.3 .5   1 1.5

Favors screening   Favors no screening

Figure 11. Pooled Analysis of Emergency Operations in One-Time Screening Trials (Random-Effects Model)

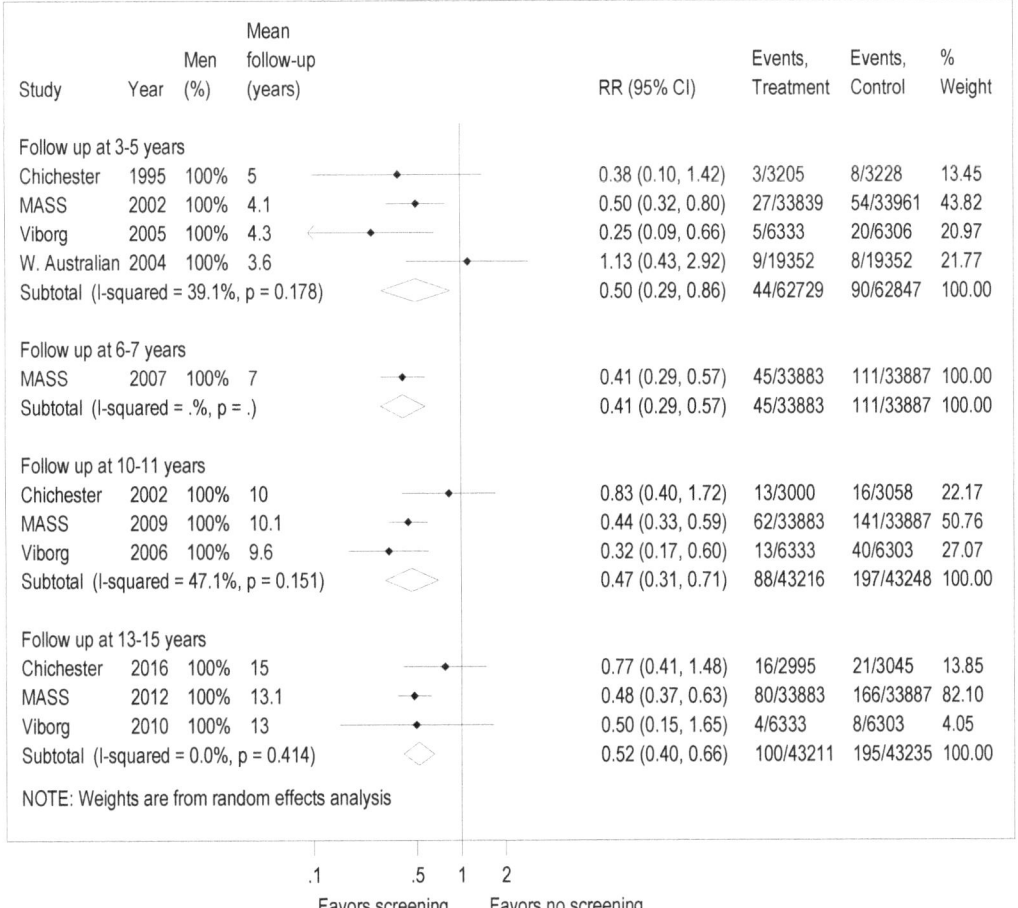

Study	Year	Men (%)	Mean follow-up (years)	RR (95% CI)	Events, Treatment	Events, Control	% Weight
Follow up at 3-5 years							
Chichester	1995	100%	5	0.38 (0.10, 1.42)	3/3205	8/3228	13.45
MASS	2002	100%	4.1	0.50 (0.32, 0.80)	27/33839	54/33961	43.82
Viborg	2005	100%	4.3	0.25 (0.09, 0.66)	5/6333	20/6306	20.97
W. Australian	2004	100%	3.6	1.13 (0.43, 2.92)	9/19352	8/19352	21.77
Subtotal (I-squared = 39.1%, p = 0.178)				0.50 (0.29, 0.86)	44/62729	90/62847	100.00
Follow up at 6-7 years							
MASS	2007	100%	7	0.41 (0.29, 0.57)	45/33883	111/33887	100.00
Subtotal (I-squared = .%, p = .)				0.41 (0.29, 0.57)	45/33883	111/33887	100.00
Follow up at 10-11 years							
Chichester	2002	100%	10	0.83 (0.40, 1.72)	13/3000	16/3058	22.17
MASS	2009	100%	10.1	0.44 (0.33, 0.59)	62/33883	141/33887	50.76
Viborg	2006	100%	9.6	0.32 (0.17, 0.60)	13/6333	40/6303	27.07
Subtotal (I-squared = 47.1%, p = 0.151)				0.47 (0.31, 0.71)	88/43216	197/43248	100.00
Follow up at 13-15 years							
Chichester	2016	100%	15	0.77 (0.41, 1.48)	16/2995	21/3045	13.85
MASS	2012	100%	13.1	0.48 (0.37, 0.63)	80/33883	166/33887	82.10
Viborg	2010	100%	13	0.50 (0.15, 1.65)	4/6333	8/6303	4.05
Subtotal (I-squared = 0.0%, p = 0.414)				0.52 (0.40, 0.66)	100/43211	195/43235	100.00

NOTE: Weights are from random effects analysis

.1   .5 1 2

Favors screening   Favors no screening

Figure 12. Pooled Analysis of All-Cause Mortality, AAA-Related Mortality, and Rupture in Open Surgery vs. Surveillance at 5-Year Followup (Random-Effects Model)

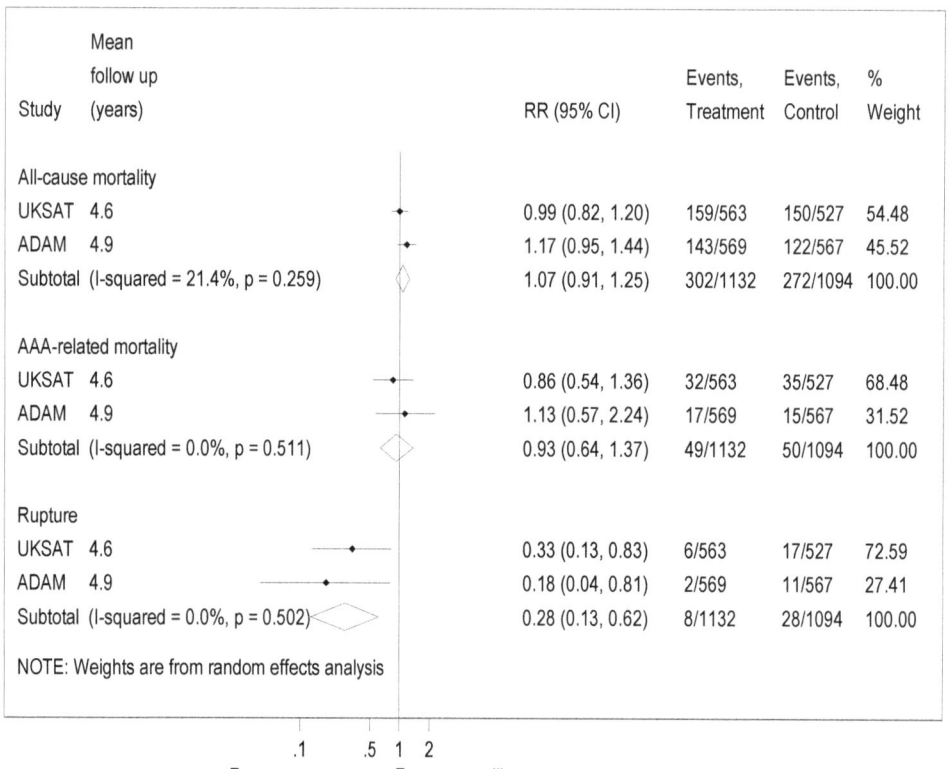

Study	Mean follow up (years)	RR (95% CI)	Events, Treatment	Events, Control	% Weight
All-cause mortality					
UKSAT	4.6	0.99 (0.82, 1.20)	159/563	150/527	54.48
ADAM	4.9	1.17 (0.95, 1.44)	143/569	122/567	45.52
Subtotal (I-squared = 21.4%, p = 0.259)		1.07 (0.91, 1.25)	302/1132	272/1094	100.00
AAA-related mortality					
UKSAT	4.6	0.86 (0.54, 1.36)	32/563	35/527	68.48
ADAM	4.9	1.13 (0.57, 2.24)	17/569	15/567	31.52
Subtotal (I-squared = 0.0%, p = 0.511)		0.93 (0.64, 1.37)	49/1132	50/1094	100.00
Rupture					
UKSAT	4.6	0.33 (0.13, 0.83)	6/563	17/527	72.59
ADAM	4.9	0.18 (0.04, 0.81)	2/569	11/567	27.41
Subtotal (I-squared = 0.0%, p = 0.502)		0.28 (0.13, 0.62)	8/1132	28/1094	100.00

NOTE: Weights are from random effects analysis

.1   .5   1   2
Favors surgery   Favors surveillance

Figure 13. Pooled Analysis of All-Cause Mortality, AAA-Related Mortality, and Rupture in EVAR vs. Surveillance Trials (Random-Effects Model)

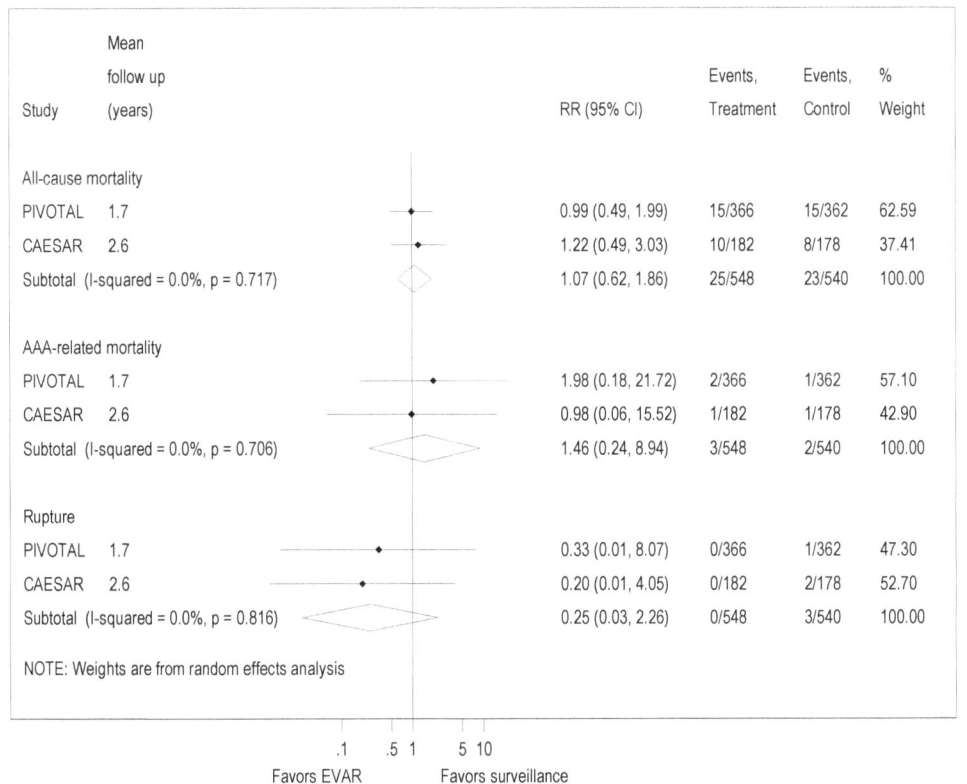

Study	Mean follow up (years)	RR (95% CI)	Events, Treatment	Events, Control	% Weight
All-cause mortality					
PIVOTAL	1.7	0.99 (0.49, 1.99)	15/366	15/362	62.59
CAESAR	2.6	1.22 (0.49, 3.03)	10/182	8/178	37.41
Subtotal (I-squared = 0.0%, p = 0.717)		1.07 (0.62, 1.86)	25/548	23/540	100.00
AAA-related mortality					
PIVOTAL	1.7	1.98 (0.18, 21.72)	2/366	1/362	57.10
CAESAR	2.6	0.98 (0.06, 15.52)	1/182	1/178	42.90
Subtotal (I-squared = 0.0%, p = 0.706)		1.46 (0.24, 8.94)	3/548	2/540	100.00
Rupture					
PIVOTAL	1.7	0.33 (0.01, 8.07)	0/366	1/362	47.30
CAESAR	2.6	0.20 (0.01, 4.05)	0/182	2/178	52.70
Subtotal (I-squared = 0.0%, p = 0.816)		0.25 (0.03, 2.26)	0/548	3/540	100.00

NOTE: Weights are from random effects analysis

.1   .5 1   5 10

Favors EVAR   Favors surveillance

Figure 14. Pooled Analysis of All-Cause Mortality in Trials of Antibiotics vs. Placebo (Random-Effects Model)

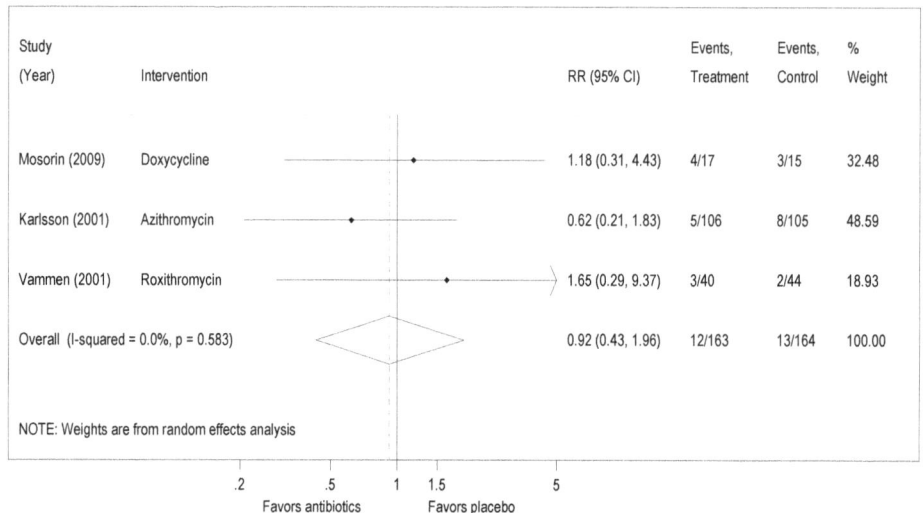

Study (Year)	Intervention	RR (95% CI)	Events, Treatment	Events, Control	% Weight
Mosorin (2009)	Doxycycline	1.18 (0.31, 4.43)	4/17	3/15	32.48
Karlsson (2001)	Azithromycin	0.62 (0.21, 1.83)	5/106	8/105	48.59
Vammen (2001)	Roxithromycin	1.65 (0.29, 9.37)	3/40	2/44	18.93
Overall (I-squared = 0.0%, p = 0.583)		0.92 (0.43, 1.96)	12/163	13/164	100.00

NOTE: Weights are from random effects analysis

Favors antibiotics   Favors placebo

Figure 15. 30-Day and Postoperative (30-Day Plus In-Hospital) Mortality in Early Open Surgery vs. Surveillance Trials (Random-Effects Model)

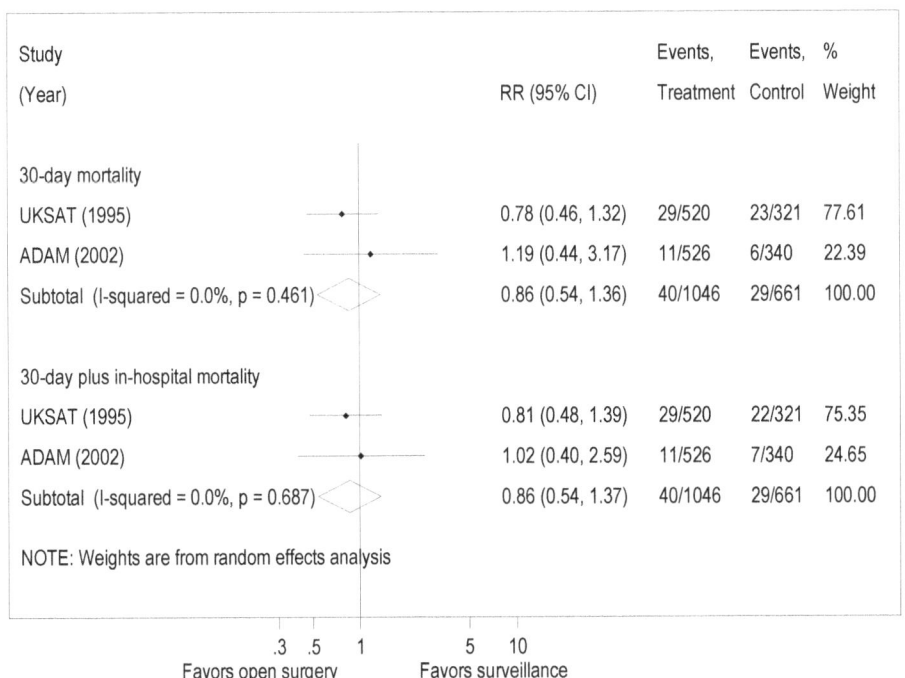

Study (Year)	RR (95% CI)	Events, Treatment	Events, Control	% Weight
30-day mortality				
UKSAT (1995)	0.78 (0.46, 1.32)	29/520	23/321	77.61
ADAM (2002)	1.19 (0.44, 3.17)	11/526	6/340	22.39
Subtotal (I-squared = 0.0%, p = 0.461)	0.86 (0.54, 1.36)	40/1046	29/661	100.00
30-day plus in-hospital mortality				
UKSAT (1995)	0.81 (0.48, 1.39)	29/520	22/321	75.35
ADAM (2002)	1.02 (0.40, 2.59)	11/526	7/340	24.65
Subtotal (I-squared = 0.0%, p = 0.687)	0.86 (0.54, 1.37)	40/1046	29/661	100.00

NOTE: Weights are from random effects analysis

.3 .5 1   5 10
Favors open surgery   Favors surveillance

* The number of events in UKSAT was estimated based on the reported proportion that was adjusted for age and sex.

Figure 16. 30-Day Operative Mortality in Early EVAR vs. Surveillance Trials

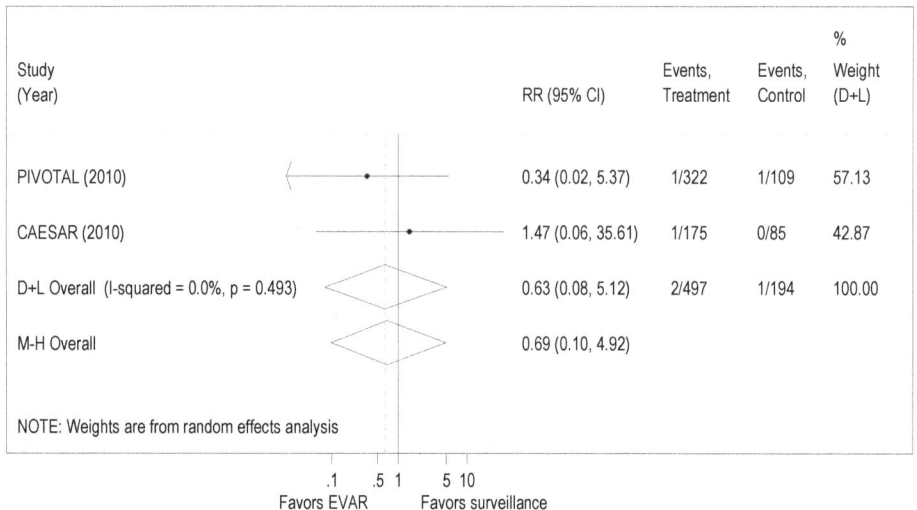

Study (Year)	RR (95% CI)	Events, Treatment	Events, Control	% Weight (D+L)
PIVOTAL (2010)	0.34 (0.02, 5.37)	1/322	1/109	57.13
CAESAR (2010)	1.47 (0.06, 35.61)	1/175	0/85	42.87
D+L Overall (I-squared = 0.0%, p = 0.493)	0.63 (0.08, 5.12)	2/497	1/194	100.00
M-H Overall	0.69 (0.10, 4.92)			

NOTE: Weights are from random effects analysis

.1 .5 1   5 10
Favors EVAR   Favors surveillance

* Both random-effect (D-L) and fixed-effect (M-H) models were included due to the very low event rates.

Table 1. AAA Prevalence, Rupture, and Surgery Data for One-Time Screening Trials (KQs 1 and 3)

Study, Year USPSTF Quality	Mean Followup, y	Treatment group	N Analyzed	AAA Prevalence, n (%)	AAA Rupture, n (%)	HR (95% CI) for AAA Rupture	All AAA Procedures, n (%)	Elective Surgery, n (%)	Emergency Surgery, n (%)	HR (95% CI) for Emergency Surgery
MASS[13,89,90] Good	4.1	IG	33,839	1,333 (4.9)*	66 (0.2)	NR	349 (1.03)	322 (0.95)	27 (0.08)	NR
		CG	33,961	NR	NR		146 (0.43)	92 (0.27)	54 (0.16)	NR
	7	IG	33,883	1,334 (4.9)	135 (0.4)	0.52 (0.42–0.64)	495 (1.5)	450 (1.3)	45 (0.13)	NR
		CG	33,887	NR	257 (0.8)		267 (0.79)	156 (0.5)	111 (0.33)	NR
	10.1	IG	33,883	1,334 (4.9)	197 (0.6)†	0.52 (0.44–0.62)	614 (1.8)	552 (1.6)	62 (0.2)	NR
		CG	33,887	NR	374 (1.1)†		367 (1.1)	226 (0.7)	141 (0.4)	NR
	13.1	IG	33,883	1,334 (4.9)	273 (0.8)	0.57 (0.49–0.66)	680 (2.0)	600 (1.8)	80 (0.2)	NR
		CG	33,887	NR	476 (1.4)		443 (1.3)	277 (0.8)	166 (0.5)	NR
Viborg[15,67,92,93] Good	4.3‡‡	IG	6,333	191 (4.0)‡	8 (0.1)	0.27 (0.13–0.60); p=0.001	53 (0.8)	48 (0.8)	5 (0.08)	0.25 (0.09–0.66); p=0.002
		CG	6,306	NR	29 (0.5)		31 (0.5)	11 (0.2)	20 (0.3)	
	5.1	IG	6,339	191 (3.9)¶	6 (0.1)	0.30 (0.11–0.78); p=0.006§	60 (0.9)	53 (0.8)	7 (0.1)	0.26 (0.10–0.62); p=0.0006§
		CG	6,319	NR	20 (0.3)		41 (0.6)	14 (0.2)	27 (0.4)	
	10	IG	6,333	NR	NR	NA	89 (1.4)	76 (1.2)	13 (0.2)	0.32 (0.17–0.60); p<0.001‖
		CG	6,306	NR	NR	NA	69 (1.1)	29 (0.5)	40 (0.6)	
	13	IG	6,333	NR	16 (0.3)	0.44 (0.24–0.79)	53 (0.8)	89 (1.4)	4 (0.06)#	0.50 (0.15–1.65)
		CG	6,306	NR	36 (0.6)		31 (0.5)	44 (0.7)	8 (0.1)#	
Chichester (men only)[14,91,124] Fair	5‡‡	IG	3,205	178 (7.6)	9 (0.3)	NR	31 (1.0)	28 (0.9)	3 (0.09)	NR
		CG	3,228	NR	20 (0.6)		13 (0.4)	5 (0.2)	8 (0.3)	
	10‡‡	IG	3,000	170 (7.7)##	Data not usable¶¶	NR	49 (1.6)	36 (1.2)	13 (0.4)	NR
		CG	3,058	NR	31 (1.0)		33 (1.1)	17 (0.6)	16 (0.5)	
	15‡‡	IG	2,995***	170†††	54 (1.8)	0.88 (0.61–1.26)	57 (1.9)	41 (1.4)	16 (0.5)	NR
		CG	3,045***	NR	63 (2.1)		40 (1.3)	19 (0.6)	21 (0.7)	
Chichester (women only)[14,25] Fair	5‡‡	IG	4,682	40 (1.3)	3 (0.06)	NR	6 (0.1)	5 (0.1)	1 (0.02)	NR
		CG	4,660	NR	3 (0.06)		NR	NR	2 (0.04)	
	10‡‡	IG	4,682	NR	10 (0.2)	NR	NR	NR	NR	NA
		CG	4,660	NR	9 (0.2)		NR	NR	NR	
Western Australian[16] Fair	3.6‡‡	IG	19,352	875 (7.2)**	33 (0.2)	NR	116 (0.6)	107 (0.5)††	9 (0.05)	NR
		CG	19,352	NR	38 (0.2)		62 (0.3)	54 (0.3)††	8 (0.04)	

* N analyzed is number screened (n=27,147) for prevalence; small (3–4.4 cm): 944 (71%); medium (4.5–5.4 cm): 223 (17%); large (≥5.5 cm): 166 (12%).
† Total incidence of rupture (deaths related to AAA plus incidence of nonfatal ruptured aneurysm).
‡ N analyzed for prevalence: 4,816.
§ OR (95% CI).
‖ RR (95% CI).
¶ N analyzed for prevalence; IG: 4,843.
# Emergency surgery without rupture.
** N analyzed for prevalence: 12,203; 3.0–4.4 cm: 699 (80%); 4.5–5.4 cm: 115 (13%); >5.4 cm: 61 (7%).

Table 1. AAA Prevalence, Rupture, and Surgery Data for One-Time Screening Trials (KQs 1 and 3)

††p=0.002.
‡‡N analyzed for prevalence: 5,394; 40 (1.3%) were in women.
§§9 in the IG were men; 20 in the CG were men.
¶¶ Due to incomplete reporting.
##N analyzed for prevalence: 2,212.
***Due to updated computer systems and the correction of data, 391 men were excluded from the original data.
†††N analyzed for prevalence: 2,216.
‡‡‡Median.

Abbreviations: AAA = abdominal aortic aneurysm; CG = control group; CI = confidence interval; HR = hazard ratio; IG = intervention group; MASS = Multicenter Aneurysm Screening Study; N = population size; n = sample size; NA = not applicable; NR = not reported.

Table 2. All-Cause and AAA-Related Mortality Data for One-Time Screening Trials (KQs 1 and 3)

Study, Year USPSTF Quality	Mean Followup, y	Treatment group	N Analyzed	All-cause mortality, n (%)	HR (95% CI)	AAA-related mortality, n (%)	HR (95% CI)
MASS[13,89,90] Good	4.1	IG	33,839	3,750 (11.1)	0.97 (0.93–1.02)	65 (0.2)*	0.58 (0.42–0.78); p=0.0002
		CG	33,961	3,855 (11.4)		113 (0.3)*	
	7	IG	33,883	6,882 (20.3)	0.96 (0.93–1.00)	105 (0.3)	0.53 (0.42–0.68); p=0.208
		CG	33,887	7,112 (21.0)		196 (0.6)	
	10.1	IG	33,883	10,274 (30.3)	0.97 (0.95–1.00)	110 (0.3)	0.52 (0.43–0.63)†
		CG	33,887	10,481 (30.9)		251 (0.7)	
	13.1	IG	33,883	13,858 (40.9)	0.97 (0.95–0.99)	224 (0.7)	0.58 (0.49–0.69)
		CG	33,887	14,134 (41.7)		381 (1.1)	
Viborg[15,67,92,93] Good	4.3¶	IG	6,333	NR	0.92 (0.84–1.00); p=0.053	9 (0.14)	0.33 (0.16–0.71); p=0.003
		CG	6,306	NR		27 (0.43)	
	5.1	IG	6,339	NR	NA	10 (0.2)	NR
		CG	6,319	NR		36 (0.6)	
	10	IG	6,333	2,184 (34)	0.97 (0.91–1.03)	14 (0.2)	0.27 (0.15–0.49); p<0.001
		CG	6,306	2,234 (35)		51 (0.8)	
	13	IG	6,333	2,931 (46.3)	0.98 (0.93–1.03)	19 (0.3)	0.34 (0.20–0.57)
		CG	6,306	2,964 (47.0)		55 (0.9)	
Chichester (men only)[14,91,124] Fair	5¶	IG	3,205	532 (16.6)	NR	10 (0.3)	NR
		CG	3,228	508 (15.7)		17 (0.5)	
	10‖¶	IG	3,000	NR	NA	24 (0.8)	0.79 (0.5–1.4)§
		CG	3,058	NR		31 (1.0)	
	15‖¶	IG	2,995‡	2,036 (68.0)	1.01 (0.95–1.07)	47 (1.6)	0.89 (0.6–1.32)
		CG	3,045‡	2,067 (67.9)		54 (1.8)	
Chichester (women only)[14,25] Fair	5¶	IG	4,682	503 (10.7)	NR	6 (0.1)	NR
		CG	4,660	476 (10.2)		2 (0.04)	
	10¶	IG	4,682	NR	NA	NR	NA
		CG	4,660	NR		NR	
Western Australian[16] Fair	3.6¶	IG	19,352	NR	NA	18 (0.09)	0.61 (0.33–1.11)§
		CG	19,352	NR		25 (0.13)	

*Defined as 30-day mortality plus deaths from ruptured AAA.
†HR includes AAA of unspecified site.
‡Due to updated computer systems and the correction of data, 391 men were excluded from the original data.
§Rate ratio (95% CI).
‖Male subgroup only.
¶Median.

Abbreviations: AAA = abdominal aortic aneurysm; CG = control group; CI = confidence interval; HR = hazard ratio; IG = intervention group; MASS = Multicenter Aneurysm Screening Study; N = population size; n = sample size; NA = not applicable; NR = not reported.

Table 3. AAA Prevalence, Rupture, and Surgery Data for Rescreening Trials (KQ 2)

Study, Year USPSTF Quality	Mean Followup, y	N Analyzed	Initial Aorta Size	AAA Incidence, n (%)	Mean Growth Rate, mm/y	AAA Rupture, n (%)	All AAA Procedures, n (%)	Elective Surgery, n (%)	Emergency Surgery, n (%)
D'Audiffret, 2002[96] Fair	5.9	223	2.5–2.9 cm	>3 cm: 141 (63) >5 cm: 3 (1.3)	1.3 ± 1.5	0	0	NA	NA
Deveraj, 2008[98] Fair	5.4	358	2.6–2.9 cm	>3 cm: 314 (88) ≥5.5 cm: 8 (2)	1.69 (1.56–1.82)	NR	NR	NR	NR
Emerton, 1994[102]	5	189	<2.5 cm	>3 cm: 2 (1.1)‖	Mean diameter unchanged, p=0.38	0	NR	NR	NR
McCarthy 2003[126] (5-year data)	5	625	2.6–2.9 cm	>5.5 cm: 2.4%	0.09 (0.02–0.17)¶	0			
Crow 2001[103] (12-year data) Darwood 2012[17]	12	129	<2.6 cm	>3 cm: 4 (3.1)	No clinically significant increase in the mean aortic diameter of participants	0	NR	NR	NR
Fair	≥10	547	2.6–2.9 cm	>4 cm: 201 (34) >5.4 cm: 87 (15)	NR	13 (2.4)	63 (11.5)	57 (9.7)	6 (1.1)
Hafez, 2008[99] Fair	5##	4,308	<3.0 cm	>3 cm: 120 (2.8)	1.8 (0.2–7.1)#	NR	NR	NR	NR
Lederle, 2000[101] Good	4	2,622	<3.0 cm	>3 cm: 58 (2.2)§§ >5 cm: 0	NR	0	0	NA	NA
Lindholt, 2000[100] Fair	5	248	2.5–2.9 cm	>3 cm: 48 (19.4) >5 cm: 0	0.5 (0.9)¶¶	NR	0	NA	NA
Scott, 2001[97] Fair	10	649	<3.0 cm	>3 cm: 27 (4.2) >5 cm: 0	NR	NR	NR	NR	NR

‖ Size distribution: 1 at 3.0 cm; 1 at 3.1 cm.
¶ Median (IQR) expansion rate for 2.6- to 2.9-cm AAA.
# Median (range).
§§ Size distribution: 3.0–3.4 cm: 45 (77.6); 3.5–3.9 cm: 10 (17.2); 4.0–4.9 cm: 3 (5.2); of these, 10 (17.2); 4.0–4.9 cm: 3 (5.2); of these, the mean initial aortic diameter was 2.3 cm. Those who did not develop an AAA had a mean aortic diameter of 2.0 cm (p<0.001).
¶¶ (SD).
Median; followup up to 10 years.

Abbreviations: AAA = abdominal aortic aneurysm; N = population size; n = sample size; NA = not applicable; NR = not reported.

Table 4. All-Cause and AAA-Related Mortality Data for Rescreening Trials (KQ 2)

Study, Year USPSTF Quality	Mean Followup, y	N Analyzed	All-cause mortality, n (%)	HR (95% CI)	AAA-related mortality, n (%)	HR (95% CI)	Operative mortality, n (%)
D'Audiffret, 2002[96] Fair	5.9	223	8 (3.6)	NR	0	NA	NR
Deveraj, 2008[98] Fair	5.4	358	NR	NA	NR	NA	NR
Emerton, 1994[102]	5	189	NR	NR	0	NR	NR
	5	625	NR		NR		
McCarthy 2003[126] (5-year data)	12	129	NR	NR	0	NR	NR
Crow 2001[103] (12-year data)	≥10	547	199 (34)	NR	14 (2.4)	NR	7 (11.1)
Darwood 2012[17] Fair							
Hafez, 2008[99] Fair	5*	4,308	NR	NA	NR	NR	NR
Lederle, 2000[101] Good	4	2,622	NR	NR	0	NR	NA
Lindholt, 2000[100] Fair	5	248	NR	NR	NR	NA	NR
Scott, 2001[97] Fair	10	649	NR	NA	NR	NR	NR

*Median.

Abbreviations: CI = confidence interval; HR = hazard ratio; N = population size; n = sample size; NA = not applicable; NR = not reported.

Table 5. AAA Growth Rate, Rupture, and Surgery Data for Open Surgery vs. Surveillance Trials for Small AAA (KQs 4 and 5)

Study, Year USPSTF Quality	Mean Followup, y	Treatment group	N Analyzed	Mean AAA Growth Rate, mm/y (IQR)	AAA Rupture, n (%)	All AAA Procedures, n (%)	Elective Surgery, n (%)	Emergency Surgery, n (%)
ADAM[106] Good	4.9	IG	569	NA	2 (0.4)	527 (92.6)	NR (92.6)	NR
		CG	567	3.2 (1.6–4.2)‡	11 (1.9)*	349 (61.6)	NR	NR
UKSAT[41,108,109] Good	4.6	IG	563	NA	6 (1.2)	520 (92.4)	517 (91.8)	3
		CG	527	3.3 (2.0–5.3)§	17 (3.2)	321 (60.9)	NR	NR
	8	IG	563	NR	10 (1.8)†	526 (92.0)	905 (83.0)	3 (0.53)
		CG	527	NR	23 (4.3)	389 (62.0)	NR	7 (1.32)
	12	IG	563	NR	13 (2.3)*	528 (93.8)	525 (93.3)	3 (0.5)
		CG	527	NR	24 (4.5)	401 (76.1)	395 (75.0)	6 (1.1)

*Deaths from ruptures, plus two additional whose group was not reported.
†Calculated from those who had emergency repair of ruptured aneurysm and survived plus those who died from rupture in both groups.
‡Average growth at 3 years.
§Median.
‖ Total elective surgeries; treatment group NR.

Abbreviations: AAA = abdominal aortic aneurysm; ADAM = Abdominal Aortic Aneurysm Detection and Management Study; CG = control group; IG = intervention group; IQR = interquartile range; N = population size; n = sample size; NA = not applicable; NR = not reported; UKSAT = U.K. Small Aneurysm Trial.

Table 6. All-Cause and AAA-Related Mortality Data for Open Surgery vs. Surveillance Trials for Small AAA (KQ 4)

Study, Year USPSTF Quality	Mean Followup, y	Treatment group	N Analyzed	All-cause mortality, n (%)	HR (95% CI)	AAA-related mortality, n (%)	HR (95% CI)
ADAM[106] Good	4.9	IG	569	143 (25.1)	1.21 (0.95 to 1.54)	17 (3.0)	1.15 (0.58 to 2.31)
		CG	567	122 (21.5)		15 (2.6)	
UKSAT[41,108,109] Good	4.6	IG	563	159 (30.6)	0.91 (0.72 to 1.16)	32 (5.7)	NR
		CG	527	150 (46.7)		35 (6.6)	
	8	IG	563	242 (43.0)	0.81 (0.68 to 0.98)	54 (9.6)	NR
		CG	527	254 (48.2)		37 (7.0)	
	12	IG	563	362 (64.3)	0.88 (0.75 to 1.02)	36 (6.9)	NR
		CG	527	352 (66.8)		50 (9.5)	

Abbreviations: AAA = abdominal aortic aneurysm; ADAM = Abdominal Aortic Aneurysm Detection and Management Study; CG = control group; CI = confidence interval; HR = hazard ratio; IG = intervention group; N = population size; n = sample size; NR = not reported; UKSAT = U.K. Small Aneurysm Trial.

Table 7. AAA Growth Rate, Rupture, and Surgery Data for EVAR vs. Surveillance Trials for Small AAA (KQs 4 and 5)

Study, Year USPSTF Quality	Mean Followup, y	Treatment group	N Analyzed	AAA Growth Rate, mm/y	AAA Rupture, n (%)	All AAA Procedures, n (%)	Elective Surgery (EVAR), n (%)	Emergency Surgery, n (%)
CAESAR[113] Fair	2.5¶	IG	182	NA	0	175 (96.2)	171 (94.0)†	NR
		CG	178	1.5*	2 (1.1)	85 (47.8)	71 (39.9)‡	NR
PIVOTAL[115] Fair	1.7	IG	366	NR	0	326 (89.1)	322 (88.9)§	NR
		CG	362		1 (0.3)	112 (30.9)	108 (30.1)‖	1 (0.3)

*Mean increase in patients who were never repaired (at time of analysis).
†4 patients (2.3%) received repair via open surgery.
‡14 patients (7.9%) received repair via open surgery.
§5 patients (1.4%) received repair via open surgery.
‖3 patients (0.8%) received repair via open surgery.
¶Median.

Abbreviations: AAA = abdominal aortic aneurysm; CAESAR = Comparison of Surveillance vs. Aortic Endografting for Small Aneurysm Repair; CG = control group; EVAR = endovascular aneurysm repair; IG = intervention group; N = population size; n = sample size; NA = not applicable; NR = not reported; PIVOTAL = Positive Impact of Endovascular Options for Treating Aneurysms Early.

Table 8. All-Cause and AAA-Related Mortality Data for EVAR vs. Surveillance Trials for Small AAA (KQ 4)

Study, Year USPSTF Quality	Mean Followup, y	Treatment group	N Analyzed	All-cause mortality, n (%)	HR (95% CI)	AAA-related mortality, n (%)	HR (95% CI)
CAESAR[113] Fair	2.6*	IG	182	10 (5.5)	0.76 (0.30 to 1.93)	1 (0.5)	NR
		CG	178	8 (4.5)		1 (0.6)	
PIVOTAL[115] Fair	1.7	IG	366	15 (4.1)	1.01 (0.49 to 2.07)	2 (0.5)	NR
		CG	362	15 (4.1)		1 (0.3)	

*Median.

Abbreviations: AAA = abdominal aortic aneurysm; CAESAR: Comparison of Surveillance vs. Aortic Endografting for Small Aneurysm Repair; CG = control group; CI = confidence interval; EVAR = endovascular aneurysm repair; HR = hazard ratio; IG = intervention group; N = population size; n = sample size; NA = not applicable; NR = not reported; PIVOTAL = Positive Impact of Endovascular Options for Treating Aneurysms Early.

Table 9. AAA Growth Rate, Rupture, and Surgery Data for Pharmacotherapy vs. Placebo Trials for Small AAA (KQs 4 and 5)

Study, Year USPSTF Quality	Comparison	Mean Followup, y	Treatment Group	N Analyzed	Mean AAA Growth Rate, mm/y	AAA Rupture, n (%)	All AAA Procedures, n (%)	Elective Surgery, n (%)	Emergency Surgery, n (%)
Mosorin 2001[118] Fair	Doxycycline vs. placebo	1.5	IG	17	1.5 (0.0–3.0)†	1 (5.9)	3 (17.6)	2 (11.8)	1 (5.9)
			CG	15	3.0 (0.3–6.0)†	0	6 (40.0)	6 (40.0)	0
Karlsson 2009[119] Fair	Azithromycin vs. placebo	1.5	IG	106	2.2 (0.12–0.36)§	1 (0.94)	16 (15.1)	15‡	1‡
			CG	105	2.2 (0.09–0.34)§	NR	13 (12.4)	NR	NR
Vammen 2001[120]	Roxithromycin vs. placebo	2	IG	40	1.56‖	NR	5 (12.5)	5 (11.6)	NR
Hogh 2009[121]			CG	44	2.75‖	NR	7 (15.9)	7 (14.3)	NR
Good		5	IG	42	1.16¶	NR	29 (34.5)#	29 (34.5)#	NR
			CG	42	2.52¶	NR			NR
PAT, 2002[116] Good	Propranolol vs. placebo	2.5	IG	276	2.1 (0.29)*	1 (0.4)	57 (20.6)	56 (20.3)	1 (0.4)
			CG	272	2.6 (0.30)*	2 (0.7)	74 (27.2)	72 (26.5)	2 (0.7)

*While patients were taking the study drug assigned; values reported as mean growth rate (SD); p=0.10.
†Median (IQR); p-value was not significant.
‡Assumed.
§Median (IQR); p=0.85.
‖p=0.02; n differed from other outcomes: IG: 32; CG: 38.
¶p=0.055.
#Total referred to surgery because AAA was >5.0 cm (treatment group NR).

Abbreviations: AAA = abdominal aortic aneurysm; CG = control group; IG = intervention group; N = population size; n = sample size; NR = not reported; PAT = Propranolol Aneurysm Trial.

Table 10. All-Cause and AAA-Related Mortality Data for Pharmacotherapy vs. Placebo Trials for Small AAA (KQ 4)

Study, Year USPSTF Quality	Comparison	Mean followup, y	Treatment group	N Analyzed	All-cause mortality, n (%)	HR (95% CI)	AAA-related mortality, n (%)	HR (95% CI)
Mosorin 2001[118] Fair	Doxycycline vs. placebo	1.5	IG	17	4 (23.5)*	NR	NR	NR
			CG	15	3 (20.0)*		NR	
Karlsson 2009[119] Fair	Azithromycin vs. placebo	1.5	IG	106	5 (4.7)	NR	0	NR
			CG	105	8 (7.6)		0	
Vammen 2001[120] Hogh 2009[121] Good	Roxithromycin vs. placebo	2	IG	40	3 (7.5)	NR	NR	NR
			CG	44	2 (4.5)		NR	
		5	IG	NR	NR	NR	NR	NR
			CG	NR	NR		NR	
PAT, 2002[116] Good	Propranolol vs. placebo	2.5	IG	57	33 (12.0)	NR	2 (0.7)	NR
			CG	74	26 (9.6)		2 (0.7)	

*Defined as being "unrelated to aneurysm."

Abbreviations: AAA = abdominal aortic aneurysm; CG = control group; CI = confidence interval; HR = hazard ratio; IG = intervention group; N = population size; n = sample size; NR = not reported; PAT = Propranolol Aneurysm Trial.

Table 11. Harms Data in Studies of Treatment for Small AAA (KQ 5)

Study	Mean Followup, y	Treatment Group	N Analyzed	30-Day Operative Mortality, n (%)	Reintervention, n (%)	Endoleak, n (%)	Readmission in 30 days, n (%)	Complication, n (%)
Open surgery vs. surveillance								
UKSAT[41,108-111]	1.0	IG	474	NR	NR	NA	30 (6.3)*	NR
		CG	NR	NR	NR	NA	NR	NR
	4.6	IG	520	30 (5.8)†	NR	NA	NR	NR
		CG	321	23 (7.1)†	NR	NA	NR	NR
	8.0	IG	526	Overall: 29 (5.5)‡ Elective: 26 Emergency: 3	NR	NA	NR	NR
		CG	389	Overall: 28 (7.2)‡ Elective: 23 Emergency: 5	NR	NA	NR	NR
	12.0	IG	526	29 (5.5)	NR	NA	NR	NR
		CG	389	29 (7.2)	NR	NA	NR	NR
ADAM[106]	4.9	IG	526	11 (2.1)	1.5% (timing or group NR)	NA	108 (20.5)§	Timing NR Any complication: 275 (52.3)‖ Major complications: MI: 5 (1.0)‖ Stroke: 3 (0.6) Pulmonary embolism: 4 (0.8) Amputation: 2 (0.4) Paraplegia: 0 Dialysis: 2 (0.6)
		CG	340	6 (1.8)		NA	56 (16.5)§	Timing NR Any complication: 193 (56.8)‖ Major complications: MI: 13 (3.8)‖ Stroke: 2 (0.6) Pulmonary embolism: 1 (0.3) Amputation: 2 (0.4) Paraplegia: 2 (0.6) Dialysis: 2 (0.6)
EVAR vs. surveillance								
CAESAR[113]	2.6§§	IG	175	1 (0.6)	10 (5.7)‖	*Within 30-days*‖¶ Type 1: 2 (1.2) Type 2: 25 (14.6) Unknown: 1 (0.6)	NR	*Within 30-days* Any morbidity related to repair: 31 (17.7)‖ Any major morbidity: 6 (3.4) Any device-related morbidity: 3 (1.7)
		CG	85	0	0‖	*Within 30-days*‖¶ Type 1: 1 (1.4) Type 2: 4 (5.6) Type 3: 1 (1.4) Unknown: 1 (1.4)	NR	*Within 30-days* Any morbidity related to repair: 5 (6.0)‖ Any major morbidity: 4 (4.7) Any device-related morbidity: NR

Table 11. Harms Data in Studies of Treatment for Small AAA (KQ 5)

Study	Mean Followup, y	Treatment Group	N Analyzed	30-Day Operative Mortality, n (%)	Reintervention, n (%)	Endoleak, n (%)	Readmission in 30 days, n (%)	Complication, n (%)
PIVOTAL[115]	1.7	IG	322	1 (0.3)	Timing NR 12 (3.7)	*Within 30-days* Overall: 36 (11.9) Type 1: 0 Type 2: 34 (11.3)	20 (4.6; group	*Within 30-days* Endograph migration: 1 (0.3) Superficial wound infection: 8 (2.5) Endograph thrombosis: 4 (1.2) Deep vein thrombosis: 1 (0.3) Serious cardiac event: 17 (5.3) Serious pulmonary event: 4 (1.2) Serious renal event: 6 (1.9)
		CG	109	1 (0.9)	Timing NR 5 (4.6)	*Within 30-days* Overall: 10 (10.3) Type 1: 1 (1.0) Type 2: 4 (9.3)	NR	*Within 30-days* Endograph migration: 0 Superficial wound infection: 1 (0.9) Endograph thrombosis: 3 (2.8) Deep vein thrombosis: 0 Serious cardiac event: 9 (8.3) Serious pulmonary event: 1 (0.9) Serious renal event: 1 (0.9)
Pharmacotherapy vs. surveillance								
Mosorin 2001[118]	1.5	IG	17	NR	NR	NR	NR	1 (5.9)#
		CG	15	NR	NR	NR	NR	1 (6.7)#
Karlsson 2009[119]	1.5	IG	106	NR	NR	NR	NR	13 (12.3)**
		CG	105	NR	NR	NR	NR	8 (7.6)**
Vammen 2001[120]	2.0	IG	40	NR	NR	NR	NR	No adverse events were reported
		CG	44	NR	NR	NR	NR	
PAT 2002[116]	2.5	IG	267	1 (1.8)††	NR	NR	NR	104 (37.7)‡‡||
		CG	272	1 (1.4)††	NR	NR	NR	58 (21.3)‡‡||
Lindholt 1999[117]	2.0	IG	30	NR	NR	NR	NR	Serious cardiac arrhythmia: 1 (3.3)‡‡ Dyspepsia: 3 (10.0)‡‡ Headache: 2 (6.7)‡‡ Dizziness: 3 (10.0)‡‡
		CG	24	NR	NR	NR	NR	Serious cardiac arrhythmia: 0‡‡ Dyspepsia: 1 (4.2)‡‡ Headache: 1 (4.2)‡‡ Dizziness: 0‡‡
Registry studies								
Golledge 2007[122]	3.2§§	NA	478	5 (1.1)	*Within 30-days* 13 (3)||	*Within 30-days* Type 1: 10 (2.1) Type 2: 35 (7.3) Type 4: 1 (0.2) 97 (20.3) patients had endoleak on followup imaging ≥30 days after procedure	NR	*Within 30-days* 52 procedural and device complications occurred in 51 (10.7) patients 72 systemic complications were noted in 64 (13.4) patients

Table 11. Harms Data in Studies of Treatment for Small AAA (KQ 5)

Study	Mean Followup, y	Treatment Group	N Analyzed	30-Day Operative Mortality, n (%)	Reintervention, n (%)	Endoleak, n (%)	Readmission in 30 days, n (%)	Complication, n (%)
Peppelenbosch 2003[123]	1.7	NA	1,962	31 (1.6)	NR	Freedom from event at 4 years Type I: Proximal: 94.7% Distal: 88.7% Type III: 85.6%	NR	Timing NR Cardiac: 55 (2.8) Pulmonary: 31 (1.6) Early procedure or device-related: 57 (2.9) 30-day systemic complications combined: 235 (12.0)

*The use of bifurcated grafts (12/30 [40%]) was associated with a 2-fold increase in the risk of reoperation; p=0.03.
†Within 2 weeks of repair, n (%): IG, 26 (5.0); CG, 18 (5.6).
‡ OR (95% CI) of postoperative death according to time of repair: 1.12 per 1-year delay (0.87 to 1.44); p=0.40.
§ Timing NR.
‖ p<0.05.
¶ Experienced an adverse event by 36 months; p<0.001.
# Discontinued the medication due to an allergic reaction.
**All patients in CG had gastrointestinal symptoms and two stopped taking medications. Three patients in IG stopped taking medications (1 due to diarrhea, 1 due to arthralgia, 1 due to allergic reaction [from antihypertension medication, not study medication]).
†† N: IG, 57; CG, 74.
‡‡ Withdrew due to complications; subset of complications. Full list of complications is in Figure 14.
§§ Median.
‖‖ Reinterventions ≤30 days after surgery; ≥30 days after surgery: 50 patients underwent 72 additional interventions by open surgery (20 times in 16 patients [5 had an EVAR procedure], EVAR (52 times in 39 patients), or combined approaches.
¶¶ Denominator is those that received EVAR: IG, 171; CG, 7; at 1 year: IG: Type 2, 19 (10.9%), Type 4: 1 (0.6%); CG: Type 2: 2 (2.4%).

Abbreviations: AAA = abdominal aortic aneurysm; ADAM = Abdominal Aortic Aneurysm Detection and Management Study; CAESAR = Comparison of Surveillance vs. Aortic Endografting for Small Aneurysm Repair; CG = control group; EVAR = endovascular aneurysm repair; IG = intervention group; MI = myocardial infarction; N = population size; n = sample size; NA = not applicable; NR = not reported; PAT = Propranolol Aneurysm Trial; PIVOTAL = Positive Impact of Endovascular Options for Treating Aneurysms Early; PVD = peripheral vascular disease; UKSAT = U.K. Small Aneurysm Trial.

Table 12. Summary of Evidence

Key Question Comparison	# of studies (k); # of observations (n)	Design Aggregate internal validity	Major limitations	Consistency	Summary of findings and precision	EPC-rated strength of evidence	Applicability
Key Question 1 (benefits of 1-time screening) 1-time invitation screening vs. no screening (men age ≥65 y)	k=4; n=137,214	4 RCTs Fair- to good-quality	Only 1 trial (MASS) reported allocation concealment; no trials reported if providers were blinded.	High: 3 trials (MASS, Chichester, Viborg) consistently found statistically significant AAA-related mortality benefit; only 1 trial (Western Australian) did not find same, but baseline population was older, with lowest adherence to screening (62.5%) and highest control group surgery rate; all trials found no all-cause mortality benefit; pooled results had low heterogeneity for all-cause mortality and greater heterogeneity for AAA-related mortality.	1-time invitation for AAA screening in men age ≥65 y reduces AAA rupture (RR, 0.27 [95% CI, 0.11 to 0.65]) at up to 10-y followup and AAA-related mortality (RR, 0.58 [95% CI, 0.39 to 0.88]) at up to 15-y followup. Screening has no effect on all-cause mortality up to 15 years in men (RR, 0.98 [95% CI, 0.97 to 1.00]).	Moderate	External validity limitations: Caucasian, male population, outside U.S. and studies did not report demographic, risk factor, or comorbidity characteristics of participants; therefore, difficult to assess if applicable to U.S. male population or how effect differs by subpopulation
Key Question 1a (subgroups) Subgroup effectiveness	Women: k=1; n=9,342 Older age: k=2; n=53,639	RCTs (1 for women, 2 for age-specific subgroup analyses) Fair-quality	Women: did not report concealment, blinding, or differential followup Age subgroup analysis: internal validity limited by nature of post-hoc subgroup analysis.	Women: N/A (only 1 study) Age: low consistency because 1 subgroup analysis (Viborg) showed older (66–73 y) and younger age (64–65 y) groups have the same AAA-related mortality benefit from screening and 1 subgroup analysis (Western Australian) showed no benefit in either older (≥75 y) or younger (65–74 y) age groups; however, populations were different in these 2 trials.	1-time AAA screening has no AAA-related or overall mortality benefit in women (based on few women studied), and no age-specific differences.	Insufficient	External validity: only 1 trial (Chichester) recruited any women (mostly Caucasian), so unclear if applicable to nonCaucasian women
Key Question 1b (screening approaches) High- vs. low-risk approach to screening	k=1; n=12,639	1 simulation from RCT N/A	Comorbidities ascertained from hospital discharge summaries (under-ascertainment), biasing against high-risk screening yield; comorbidity information collected post-randomization, thereby making this study a simulation.	N/A (only 1 study)	High- vs. low-risk approach: involves a tradeoff but absolute yield cannot be determined because of a lack of RCT-level or large generalizable cohort.	Insufficient	Concerns about internal validity make external validity unclear

Table 12. Summary of Evidence

Key Question Comparison	# of studies (k); # of observations (n)	Design Aggregate internal validity	Major limitations	Consistency	Summary of findings and precision	EPC-rated strength of evidence	Applicability
Key Question 2 (benefits of repeated screening)	k=8; n=11,583	6 cohorts, 1 case-control, 1 patient-level meta-analysis Fair-quality	All were underpowered to detect AAA-related mortality difference and 3 studies reported no AAA-related mortality rates; therefore, growth rate/AAA incidence (intermediate outcomes) were the focus of results. Sparse demographic/risk factor information: only 2 studies reported this (both from ADAM subset). All studies had no adjustment for confounders. Only ADAM subset trial included women.	Too heterogeneous: rescreening interval frequently varied; no participant characteristics reported to understand if the populations were comparable; likely baseline characteristics of participants or imaging approaches were quite different across studies, as reflected by a wide variation in AAA incidence (2% to 88% initially normal aortas developed AAA ≥3 cm at 5-y followup). The patient-level meta-analysis reported a mean time from presentation to AAA rupture of 18.7 y.	Insufficient information for firm conclusions about yield of rescreening.	Low	Unclear: no population demographic/risk factor information for 5 out of 7 studies; 2 studies were in U.S.; most studies in men only
Key Question 2a (subgroups) Subgroup effectiveness	k=2; n=2,845	2 cohorts (both subsets from ADAM trial) Fair-quality	Studies did not report blinding or loss to followup. No adjustment for confounders was reported.	Inconsistent: both studies are subsets from same ADAM trial; smaller study found no association between risk factors tested and AAA incidence, larger study found associations using multilogistic regression with 3 factors (smoking, CAD, any atherosclerosis).	Conclusions about yield of rescreening by age, risk factor, or comorbidity limited by small number of events; conclusions about race and sex subgroups not possible because studies almost exclusively recruited white males; imprecise findings from the same study, perhaps due to power.	Low	VA populations, mostly men, so unclear if generalizable to greater U.S. population

Table 12. Summary of Evidence

Key Question Comparison	# of studies (k); # of observations (n)	Design Aggregate internal validity	Major limitations	Consistency	Summary of findings and precision	EPC-rated strength of evidence	Applicability
Key Question 2b (screening interval)	k=8; n=11,583	6 prospective cohorts; 1 case-control; 1 patient-level meta-analysis Poor-quality: studies highly heterogeneous, all studies underpowered to detect health outcomes	See details for KQ 2.	See details for KQ 2.	Insufficient information for conclusions about yield of rescreening by frequency.	Insufficient	See KQ 2 details
Key Question 3 (harms of screening)	Operative mortality and surgery: k=4; n=137,214 QOL: k=4; n=1,333	4 RCTs (operative mortality) Fair- to good-quality 5 observational studies (QOL) Poor-quality	Operative mortality/surgery: no major concerns of internal validity. QOL: small, pre-post studies, all self-administered questionnaires; no adjustment for confounders.	Operative mortality/surgery: consistent QOL: while heterogeneous designs, followup, and possibly populations (no baseline characteristics reported), overall studies consistently show no long-term QOL differences.	Invitation for screening is associated with more overall surgeries, more elective surgeries, and fewer emergent repairs up to 15-y followup; fewer emergency operations up to 10.1 y; lower 30-day operative mortality up to 10.1 y; no long-term difference in QOL, although screen-positive patients may have statistically lower short-term QOL at 6 weeks, which does not persist.	Operative mortality/ surgery: high QOL: low	Operative mortality/surgery: community surgeons, although outside U.S., likely applicable. QOL: unclear: no population demographic/risk factor information reported
Key Question 4 (benefits of treatment) Early open surgery vs. surveillance for small AAA	k=2; n=2,226	2 RCTs Good-quality	Both good-quality internal validity. UKSAT did not report AAA mortality or rupture as primary or secondary outcomes, so ascertainment method not described.	Consistent results in both trials. There were some differences in baseline population characteristics between the 2 trials; UKSAT had less HTN, CAD, and DM, but even with these differences, consistent results of no AAA-related mortality, rupture, or all-cause mortality benefit with early open surgery were seen in both trials.	Early surgery compared with surveillance for small AAA (4 to 5 cm) decreases AAA rupture (RR, 0.28 [95% CI, 0.13–0.62]) with attenuated benefit after 5 y, but does not alter all-cause or AAA-related mortality at 5-, 8-, or 12-y followup.	High	1 trial was in the VA system, so possibly older population with more comorbidities, could influence surgical outcomes

Table 12. Summary of Evidence

Key Question Comparison	# of studies (k); # of observations (n)	Design Aggregate internal validity	Major limitations	Consistency	Summary of findings and precision	EPC-rated strength of evidence	Applicability
Key Question 4 (benefits of treatment) EVAR vs. surveillance for small AAA	k=2; n=1,088	2 RCTs Fair-quality	Internal validity: industry sponsored, stopped early for futility so randomized groups were not similar for family history, sex, or DM.	Consistent results for all studies: no difference in all-cause or AAA-related mortality.	Early EVAR compared with surveillance for small AAA (4.0 to 5.0 or 5.4 cm) does not reduce all-cause mortality, AAA-related mortality, or AAA rupture.	Moderate	PIVOTAL participants had more comorbidities and higher risk than CAESAR and perhaps more comorbidities/ higher risks than general population: family history of AAA (25%), higher CAD (55%), higher smoking (91%) proportion; therefore, may represent higher risk, especially with such high proportion with family history
Key Question 4 (benefits of treatment) Pharmacotherapy vs. placebo for small AAA	Antibiotics: k=3; n=371 Propranolol: k=1; n=552	5 RCTs Fair-quality	Small trials with primary outcome of AAA-growth; underpowered to detect health outcomes.	Inconsistent results: 4 trials each tested a different drug with heterogeneous baseline populations (different risks, sex). Some suggest decrease in AAA growth, others do not.	Short treatment with antibiotics (doxycycline, azithromycin, and roxithromycin) and beta-blocker (propranolol) does not appear to reduce AAA growth. Studies underpowered to conclude effect on health outcomes (AAA-related and all-cause mortality).	Low	Recruited from vascular center referrals, screening programs; difficult to make conclusions about generalizability because of single studies
Key Question 4a (subgroups) Subgroup effectiveness for treatment of small AAA	Open repair vs. surveillance: k=2; n=2,226 No subgroup results reported for EVAR or pharmacotherapy	2 RCTs	Few women in ADAM; no results reported by smoking history, family history, comorbidity, or race in either RCT.	RCTs showed no all-cause mortality by age or AAA diameter. Only 1 trial with women.	At 5 y, no subgroup differences in all-cause mortality by age, sex, or AAA diameter. No evidence regarding smoking history, family history, comorbidity, or race subgroup differences.		1 trial (ADAM) is in VA population; largely older, male, multiple comorbid population compared with general population

Table 12. Summary of Evidence

Key Question Comparison	# of studies (k); # of observations (n)	Design Aggregate internal validity	Major limitations	Consistency	Summary of findings and precision	EPC-rated strength of evidence	Applicability
Key Question 5 (harms of treatment) Early open surgery vs. surveillance for small AAA	Medical health outcomes/ complications: k=2; n= 2,226 QOL: k=2; n=2,001	2 RCTs (health complications) Fair-quality 2 RCTs (QOL) Fair-quality	Small number of complications in each group.	Consistent complications and 30-day postoperative mortality.	Number of operations higher in early surgery group than surveillance group. Total major complications and MI more common in surveillance group compared than early surgery group, but 30-day postoperative mortality same in both groups. Health perception/overall health was improved in those undergoing early open surgery in first 1 to 2 y after discovery, but no difference in overall QOL between surgery and surveillance groups.	Moderate	ADAM trial was conducted in VA population, so question of applicability as high prevalence of coronary disease and overall sicker patients than general older male (>50 y) population
Key Question 5 (harms of treatment) Early EVAR vs. surveillance for small AAA	Health complications: k=4; n=2,440 QOL: k=1; n=339	2 RCTs, 2 registries (health complications) Fair-quality 1 RCT (QOL) Fair-quality	Industry sponsored, few harm events because RCTs were small trials, which were stopped prematurely because of futility.	Registries consistent in systemic complications. Higher 30-day postoperative mortality in EVAR reported in registries compared with PIVOTAL or CAESAR trials.	EVAR complications: systemic complications with EVAR approximately 15%. Endoleaks approximately 10%. Reintervention approximately 4%. Operative mortality does not appear to be different for early vs. late EVAR, suggesting that delay does not lead to poorer surgical outcomes. QOL better in early EVAR vs. surveillance group in the first 6 mo post-randomization, but no difference at 3 y.	Moderate	Registries likely closer to community practice complication rates and underlying population risk

Table 12. Summary of Evidence

Key Question Comparison	# of studies (k); # of observations (n)	Design Aggregate internal validity	Major limitations	Consistency	Summary of findings and precision	EPC-rated strength of evidence	Applicability
Key Question 5 (harms of treatment) Pharmacotherapy vs. placebo for small AAA	Propranolol: k=2; n=606 Antibiotics: k=3; n=371	2 RCTs (propranolol) Fair-quality 3 RCTs (antibiotics) Poor-quality	All small trials	Propanol RCTs show a consistent lack of tolerability with no benefit. Antibiotic trials: heterogeneous; only 1 study for each antibiotic; making broad conclusions about antibiotics by qualitatively combining these studies not clinically appropriate.	Propranolol poorly tolerated, causing high withdrawal rate. Few adverse reactions reported in antibiotics studies but few events overall due to small number of participants.	Insufficient to low	Unclear

Abbreviations: AAA = abdominal aortic aneurysm; ADAM = Abdominal Aortic Aneurysm Detection and Management Study; CAD = coronary artery disease; CAESAR = Comparison of Surveillance vs. Aortic Endografting for Small Aneurysm Repair; CI = confidence interval; DM = diabetes mellitus; EPC = Evidence-based Practice Center; EVAR = endovascular aneurysm repair; HTN = hypertension; KQ = key question; MASS = Multicenter Aneurysm Screening Study; MI = myocardial infarction; N/A = not applicable; PIVOTAL = Positive Impact of Endovascular Options for Treating Aneurysms Early; QOL = quality of life; RCT = randomized, controlled trial; RR = relative risk; UKSAT = U.K. Small Aneurysm Trial; VA = Department of Veterans Affairs.

Table 13. Odds Ratios of Risk Factors Associated With Developing AAA (Based on Adjusted Multivariate Analyses)

Factors associated with AAA	Any AAA ≥3 cm[157]	Any AAA ≥4 cm[48]	Any AAA ≥5 cm[158]
Male sex (vs. female sex)	5.71	NR	7.70
Female sex (vs. male sex)	NR	0.22	NR
Age (vs. <55 y)	////////////	1.65	////////////
55–59	2.76	////////////	3.20
60–64	5.35	////////////	8.10
65–69	9.41	////////////	13.20
70–74	14.46	////////////	20.70
75–79	20.43	////////////	32.0
≥80	28.37	////////////	53.10
Hispanic/black/Asian (vs. white)	0.69 to 0.72	0.49 to 0.91	0.70
Family history of AAA	3.80	1.95	3.20
Smoking: years (<10 y, 10 to 35 y or >35 y) + packs per day (≤0.5, 0.5 to 1, >1)	2.61 to 12.13	5.57	2.60 to 14.50
Smoking cessation (5 to 10 y, >10 y)	0.42 to 0.87	NR	0.50 to 0.80
Diabetes	0.75	0.54	0.70
CVD morbidity	1.1 to 1.7	0.67 to 1.62	1.10 to 1.70

Abbreviations: AAA = abdominal aortic aneurysm; CVD = cardiovascular disease; NR = not reported.

Appendix A Table 1. Inclusion/Exclusion Criteria

Category	Inclusion	Exclusion
Populations	One-time and repeated screening (KQs 1–3): Asymptomatic adult population Treatment of small AAA (KQs 4, 5): Asymptomatic adult population with small AAA (3.0–5.4 cm)	One-time and repeated screening (KQs 1–3): Patients experiencing symptoms related to AAA Treatment of Small AAA (KQs 4, 5): Patients experiencing symptoms related to AAA, populations with AAA >5.4 cm or <3.0 cm
Setting	Conducted in primary care or other setting with primary care–comparable population Countries applicable to U.S. (all countries listed as "very high" on the Human Development Index)	
Disease/ Condition	Abdominal aortic aneurysm (aortic diameter ≥3.0 cm)	
Screening	Ultrasound	Physical examination, CT, MRI
Treatment/ management interventions or exposure	One-time and repeated screening (KQs 1–3): General or targeted screening with ultrasound Targeted screening may include the following: • Screening based on one or more risk factors • Screening based on risk derived from prediction/prognostic modeling) Treatment of small AAA (KQs 4, 5): Pharmacotherapy (statins, ACEIs, beta-blockers, antibiotics), surgery (open and EVAR), surveillance	One-time screening (KQ 1): Repeat AAA screening Repeat screening (KQ 2): One-time AAA screening
Comparisons or nonexposure	One-time screening (KQ 1): No screening, comparison of different screening approaches Repeat screening (KQ 2): No screening or one-time AAA screening using ultrasound, different repeated screening approaches, or no comparison/nonexposure Treatment of small AAA (KQs 4, 5): Surveillance, usual care, or placebo	Comparative effectiveness of treatments (KQs 4, 5)

Appendix A Table 1. Inclusion/Exclusion Criteria

Category	Inclusion	Exclusion

Outcomes	Effectiveness of one-time and repeated screening (KQs 1, 2): All-cause mortality, AAA-related mortality, AAA rupture rate, AAA incidence (KQ 2 only)
	
	Harms of screening (KQ 3): Anxiety from risk labeling, anxiety of mortality, false-positive screening-related procedure, operative mortality, surgical procedures, and quality of life
	
	Effectiveness of treatment of small AAA (KQ 4): AAA annual growth rate, all-cause mortality, AAA-related mortality, operative mortality, AAA rupture rate, and quality of life
	
	Harms of treatment of small AAA (KQ 5):
	Surgery:
	• Operative mortality
	• Cardiac and vascular complications (e.g., MI, heart failure, arrhythmia, and stroke)
	• Pulmonary complications (e.g., respiratory distress, pneumonia)
	• Renal complications (e.g., renal failure, renal vein fistula, impaired renal function postsurgery)
	• Nerve system complications (e.g., impairment of sexual function)
	• Gastrointestinal complications (e.g., aortoenteric fistulas)
	• Blood loss
	• Infection (e.g., sepsis)
	• Readmission to hospital within 30 days
	• Time for recovery
	• EVAR-specific complications:
	  ○ Device migration
	  ○ Graft thrombosis (e.g., lower limb thrombosis)
	  ○ Kinking of device
	  ○ Conversion to open surgery
	  ○ Reinterventions
	  ○ Endoleak (any type)
	Pharmacotherapy: Serious adverse events (e.g., cognitive loss, muscle breakdown, neuropathy, pancreatic and hepatic dysfunction, sexual dysfunction), discontinuation of treatment
	Surveillance: Anxiety from risk labeling, anxiety of mortality	

Study Designs	Effectiveness of screening, one-time and repeated (KQs 1, 2): RCTs, CCTs, large cohort studies (n>1,000, KQ 2 only) Effectiveness of treatment of small AAA (KQ 4): RCTs, SERs Harms of screening or treatment (KQ 3, 5): RCTs, cohort studies, case-control studies (KQ 3), SERs, registries	Effectiveness of screening, one-time and repeated (KQs 1, 2): Case-control and cross-sectional studies, editorial, letter, nonsystematic review, opinion, cost studies Effectiveness of treatment of small AAA (KQ 4): Cohort and case-control study, cross-sectional study, editorial, letter, nonsystematic review, opinion, cost studies Harms of screening or treatment (KQs 3, 5): Case-control (KQ 5), editorial, letter, nonsystematic review, opinion, cost studies
Language	English only	NonEnglish languages
Quality	Fair- and good-quality studies	Poor-quality studies

Appendix B. Search Strategies

Screening for abdominal aortic aneurysm
Search strategies (updated 1/31/2013)

Databases searched:
MEDLINE
PubMed
Cochrane Central Register of Controlled Trials
Cochrane Database of Systematic Reviews
Database of Abstracts of Reviews of Effects

Key:
/ = MeSH subject heading
* = truncation
ti = word in title
ab = word in abstract
pt = publication type
sb = subset

MEDLINE: screening
Ovid MEDLINE(R), Ovid MEDLINE(R) Daily Update
1 Aortic Aneurysm, Abdominal/
2 abdominal aortic aneurysm*.ti,ab.
3 1 or 2
4 Mass Screening/
5 Screen*.ti,ab.
6 4 or 5
7 3 and 6
8 limit 7 to (english language and yr="2004 -Current")

MEDLINE: clinical trials
Ovid MEDLINE(R), Ovid MEDLINE(R) Daily Update
1   Aortic Aneurysm, Abdominal/
2   abdominal aortic aneurysm*.ti,ab.
3   1 or 2
4   clinical trials as topic/ or controlled clinical trials as topic/ or randomized controlled trials as topic/
5   (clinical trial or controlled clinical trial or meta analysis or randomized controlled trial).pt.
6   random*.ti,ab.
7   control groups/ or double-blind method/ or single-blind method/
8   clinical trial*.ti,ab.
9   controlled trial*.ti,ab.
10 4 or 5 or 6 or 7 or 8 or 9
11 3 and 10
limit 11 to (english language and yr="2004 -Current")

MEDLINE: treatment cohort studies
Ovid MEDLINE(R), Ovid MEDLINE(R) Daily Update
1 Aortic Aneurysm, Abdominal/co, dt, mo, pc, px, rh, su, th [Complications, Drug Therapy, Mortality, Prevention & Control, Psychology, Rehabilitation, Surgery, Therapy]
2 cohort studies/ or longitudinal studies/ or follow-up studies/ or prospective studies/ or retrospective studies/
3 cohort*.ti,ab.
4 2 or 3
5 1 and 4
6 limit 5 to (english language and yr="2004 -Current")

MEDLINE: all key questions
Ovid MEDLINE(R) In-Process & Other Non-Indexed Citations
1   abdominal aortic aneurysm*.ti,ab.
2   screen*.ti,ab.

Appendix B. Search Strategies

3   random*.ti,ab.
4   clinical trial*.ti,ab.
5   controlled trial*.ti,ab.
6   cohort*.ti,ab.
7   longitudinal*.ti,ab.
8   follow up.ti,ab.
9   prospective*.ti,ab.
10   retrospective*.ti,ab.
11   meta analys*.ti,ab.
12   metaanalys*.ti,ab.
13   2 or 3 or 4 or 5 or 6 or 7 or 8 or 9 or 10 or 11 or 12
14   1 and 13
15   limit 14 to (english language and yr="2004 -Current")

PubMed: all key questions, publisher-supplied non-indexed citations only
#1 "abdominal aortic aneurysm" OR "abdominal aortic aneurysms"
#2 #1 AND publisher[sb]
#3 screen*[tiab] OR trial[tiab] OR trials[tiab] OR random*[tiab] OR cohort*[tiab] OR longitudinal*[tiab] OR "follow up"[tiab] OR "followed up"[tiab] OR followup*[tiab] OR prospective*[tiab] OR retrospective*[tiab]
#4 #2 AND #3 Limits: English, Publication Date from 2004 to 3000

PubMed: systematic reviews
#1 Aortic Aneurysm, Abdominal"[Mesh] AND systematic[sb]
#2 ("abdominal aortic aneurysm"[ti] OR "abdominal aortic aneurysms"[ti]) AND systematic[sb] AND (in process[sb] OR publisher[sb] OR pubmednotmedline[sb])
#3 #1 OR #2 English, Publication Date from 2004 to 3000

Database of Abstracts of Reviews of Effects
(abdominal aortic aneurysm) OR (abdominal aortic aneurysms) IN DARE FROM 2004 TO 2013

Cochrane Central Register of Controlled Trials
"abdominal aortic aneurysm" or "abdominal aortic aneurysms", from 2004 to 2013 in Trials

Appendix B Figure 1. Literature Flow Diagram

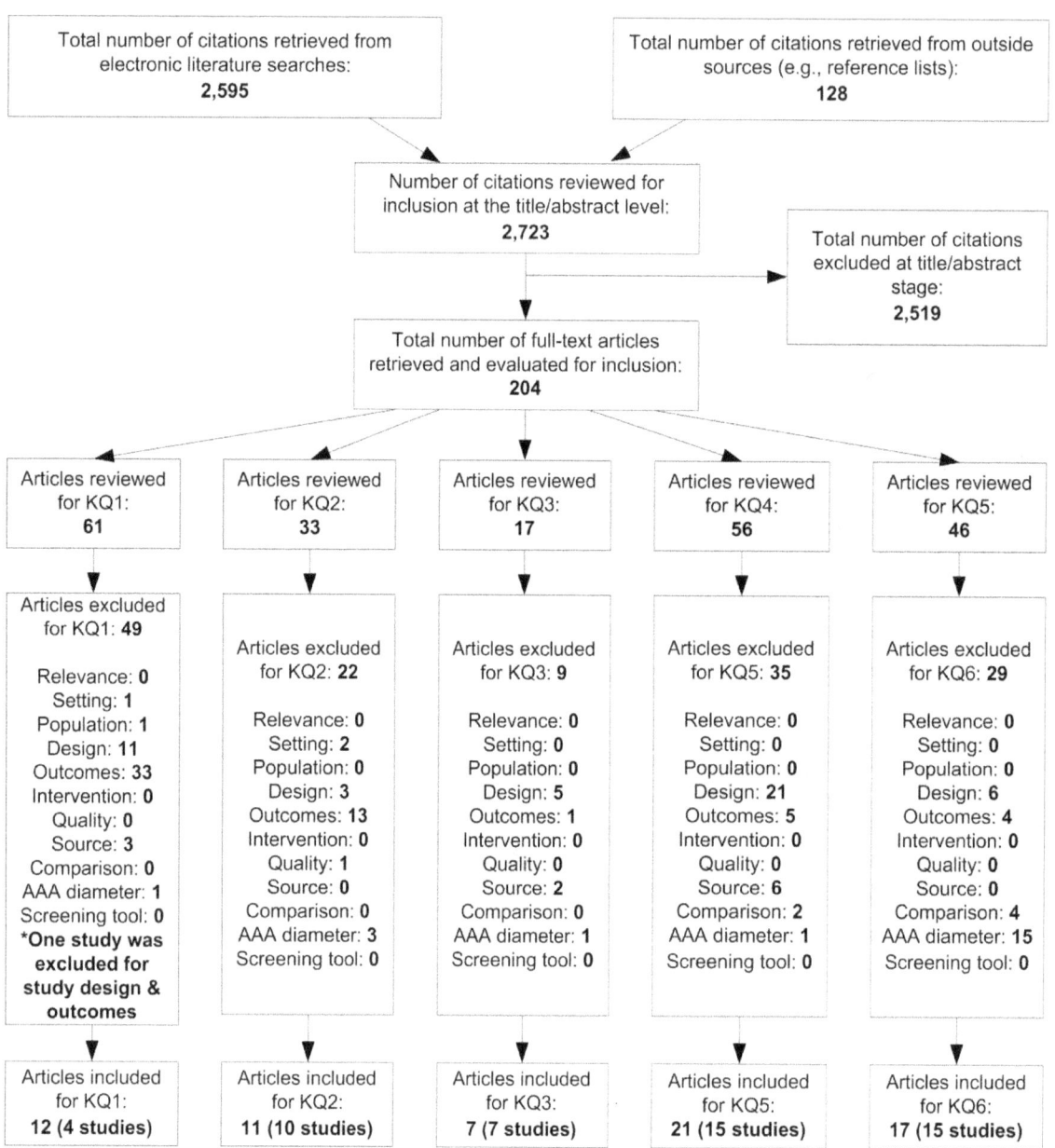

Total number of citations retrieved from electronic literature searches: **2,595**

Total number of citations retrieved from outside sources (e.g., reference lists): **128**

Number of citations reviewed for inclusion at the title/abstract level: **2,723**

Total number of citations excluded at title/abstract stage: **2,519**

Total number of full-text articles retrieved and evaluated for inclusion: **204**

Articles reviewed for KQ1: **61**

Articles reviewed for KQ2: **33**

Articles reviewed for KQ3: **17**

Articles reviewed for KQ4: **56**

Articles reviewed for KQ5: **46**

Articles excluded for KQ1: **49**

Relevance: **0**
Setting: **1**
Population: **1**
Design: **11**
Outcomes: **33**
Intervention: **0**
Quality: **0**
Source: **3**
Comparison: **0**
AAA diameter: **1**
Screening tool: **0**
*One study was excluded for study design & outcomes

Articles excluded for KQ2: **22**

Relevance: **0**
Setting: **2**
Population: **0**
Design: **3**
Outcomes: **13**
Intervention: **0**
Quality: **1**
Source: **0**
Comparison: **0**
AAA diameter: **3**
Screening tool: **0**

Articles excluded for KQ3: **9**

Relevance: **0**
Setting: **0**
Population: **0**
Design: **5**
Outcomes: **1**
Intervention: **0**
Quality: **0**
Source: **2**
Comparison: **0**
AAA diameter: **1**
Screening tool: **0**

Articles excluded for KQ5: **35**

Relevance: **0**
Setting: **0**
Population: **0**
Design: **21**
Outcomes: **5**
Intervention: **0**
Quality: **0**
Source: **6**
Comparison: **2**
AAA diameter: **1**
Screening tool: **0**

Articles excluded for KQ6: **29**

Relevance: **0**
Setting: **0**
Population: **0**
Design: **6**
Outcomes: **4**
Intervention: **0**
Quality: **0**
Source: **0**
Comparison: **4**
AAA diameter: **15**
Screening tool: **0**

Articles included for KQ1: **12 (4 studies)**

Articles included for KQ2: **11 (10 studies)**

Articles included for KQ3: **7 (7 studies)**

Articles included for KQ5: **21 (15 studies)**

Articles included for KQ6: **17 (15 studies)**

Appendix C Table 1. Ongoing Studies and Trials Pending Assessment

Investigator, study name	Location	Number of participants	Intervention	Outcomes	2013 Status
AARDVARK (Evaluation of Effect of Angiotensin-Converting Enzyme [ACE] Inhibitors on Small Aneurysm Growth Rate)	Imperial College London	225	Drug: perindopril arginine (10 mg per day) Drug: amlodipine (5 mg per day) Drug: placebo	Primary: AAA growth rate of small aneurysms (3.5–4.9 cm) measured by CTA Secondary: AAA-related mortality	Pending: Currently recruiting participants Estimated study completion date: October 2014
Grondal VIVA	Central Denmark	50,000 men	Combination AAA, PAD, and HTN screening	Primary: All-cause mortality Secondary: AAA-related mortality, AAA progression, cost, QOL	Recruitment: 2008–2010 Results pending: 3-, 5-, 10-, and 15-year followup
Smiseth	Oslo	1,500 men	Annual screening for AAA and PAD using ultrasound and AAI	Primary: AAA incidence (≥3.0 cm) Secondary: PAD incidence (measured by AAI)	Recruitment: Began January 2011 Estimated study completion date: December 2029
Dalman Study of the Effectiveness of Telmisartan in Slowing the Progression of Abdominal Aortic Aneurysms (TEDY)	U.S.	40	Drug: telmisartan (40 mg once a day) Drug: placebo	Primary: AAA growth rate of small aneurysms (3.5–4.9 cm) measured by CTA Secondary: Change in circulating AAA-biomarkers, QOL	Recruitment: Began September 2012 Estimated study completion date: August 2015
Sillesen CRD007 for the Treatment of Abdominal Aorta Aneurysm (AORTA Trial)	Denmark, Sweden, U.K.	NR	Drug: 3 dose levels of CRD007: 10, 25, and 40 mg Drug: placebo	NR	Study is completed: "no details reported"
Blankensteijn Study on Anti-inflammatory Effect of Anti-Hypertensive Treatment in Patients With Small AAA and Mild Hypertension (PISA)	The Netherlands	12	Drug: aliskiren (150–300 mg per day) Drug: amlodipine (5–10 mg per day)	Primary: change in aneurysmal vessel wall inflammation measured by PET-CT Secondary: AAA growth rate, change in large vessel inflammation	Recruitment: Began September 2011 Estimated study completion date: September 2013
Non-Invasive Treatment of Abdominal Aortic Aneurysm Clinical Trial	US	248	Drug: doxycycline (100 mg, twice a day) Drug: placebo	Primary: AAA growth rate measured by CT Secondary: Change in circulating AAA biomarkers	Recruitment: Began January 2013 Estimated study completion date: June 2017
Saiki	Japan	40	Drug: telmisartan (dose NR) Drug: placebo	Primary: AAA-growth rate	Recruitment: Began March 2010 Estimated study completion date: NR

Appendix D. Excluded Studies

Exclusion
E1. Study relevance
E2. Setting
E3. Population
E4. Study design a. Not an included study design b. Comparative effectiveness trial
E5. No relevant outcomes
E6. Interventions
E7. Study quality a. High or differential attrition b. Other issues
E8. Source document only
E9. Not relevant comparison
E10. Not relevant AAA diameter
E11. Not relevant screening tool

1. Multicentre aneurysm screening study (MASS): cost effectiveness analysis of screening for abdominal aortic aneurysms based on four year results from randomised controlled trial. BMJ 2002 Nov 16;325(7373):1135. PMID: 12433761. **KQ3E5.**

2. Abdul-Hussien H, Hanemaaijer R, Verheijen JH, et al. Doxycycline therapy for abdominal aneurysm: Improved proteolytic balance through reduced neutrophil content. J Vasc Surg 2009;49(3):741-9. PMID: 19268776. **KQ4E10.**

3. Alcorn HG, Wolfson SK, Jr., Sutton-Tyrrell K, et al. Risk factors for abdominal aortic aneurysms in older adults enrolled in The Cardiovascular Health Study. Arterioscler Thromb Vasc Biol 1996 Aug;16(8):963-70. PMID: 8696960. **KQ1E5.**

4. Ali ZA, Callaghan CJ, Ali AA, et al. Perioperative myocardial injury after elective open abdominal aortic aneurysm repair predicts outcome. Eur J Vasc Endovasc Surg 2008 Apr;35(4):413-9. PMID: 18063394. **KQ5E9.**

5. Alund M, Mani K, Wanhainen A. Selective screening for abdominal aortic aneurysm among patients referred to the vascular laboratory. Eur J Vasc Endovasc Surg 2008 Jun;35(6):669-74. PMID: 18258461. **KQ1E5.**

6. Armstrong PA, Back MR, Bandyk DF, et al. Optimizing compliance, efficiency, and safety during surveillance of small abdominal aortic aneurysms. J Vasc Surg 2007;46(2):190-5. PMID: 17540533. **KQ5E4.**

7. Arrington S, Ogata T, Davis PM, Jr., et al. Aneurysm Outreach Inc., a nonprofit organization, offers community-based, ultrasonography screening for abdominal aortic aneurysms. Ann N Y Acad Sci 2006 Nov;1085:291-3. PMID: 17182945. **KQ1E5.**

8. Badger SA, O'Donnell ME, Sharif MA, et al. Advantages and pitfalls of abdominal aortic aneurysm screening in high-risk patients. Vascular 2008 Jul;16(421):201-6. PMID: 18845100. **KQ1E4, KQ1E5, KQ2E4.**

9. Badger SA, O'Donnell ME, Sharif MA, et al. Risk factors for abdominal aortic aneurysm and the influence of social deprivation. Angiology 2008 Oct;59(5):559-66. PMID: 18818237. **KQ1E5.**

10. Bailey MA, Dunne JA, Griffin KJ, et al. Systematic review and meta-analysis of the effects of statin therapy on abdominal aortic aneurysms (Br J Surg 2011; 98: 362-353). Br J Surg 2011 May;98(5):744-5. PMID: 21462179. **KQ4E4a.**

11. Ballard DJ, Filardo G, Fowkes G, et al. Surgery for small asymptomatic abdominal aortic aneurysms. Cochrane Database Syst Rev 2008(4):CD001835. PMID: 18843626. **KQ4E8.**

12. Bartoli MA, Thevenin B, Sarlon G, et al. Secondary procedures after infrarenal abdominal aortic aneurysms endovascular repair with second-generation endografts. Ann Vasc Surg 2012 Feb;26(2):166-74. PMID: 22037143. **KQ5E10.**

13. Basnyat PS, Aiono S, Warsi AA, et al. Natural history of the ectatic aorta. Cardiovasc Surg 2003 Aug;11(4):273-6. PMID: 12802262. **KQ2E5.**

14. Baxter BT, Pearce WH, Waltke EA, et al. Prolonged administration of doxycycline in patients with small asymptomatic abdominal aortic aneurysms: report of a prospective (Phase II) multicenter study. J Vasc Surg 2002 Jul;36(1):1-12. PMID: 12096249. **KQ4E4a.**

15. Bengtsson H, Bergqvist D, Ekberg O, et al. A population based screening of abdominal aortic aneurysms (AAA). Eur J Vasc Surg 1991 Feb;5(1):53-7. PMID: 2009986. **KQ1E4a.**

Appendix D. Excluded Studies

16. Bergqvist D. Pharmacological interventions to attenuate the expansion of abdominal aortic aneurysm (AAA) - a systematic review. Eur J Vasc Endovasc Surg 2011 May;41(5):663-7. PMID: 21330159. **KQ4E8.**

17. Bertero C, Carlsson P, Lundgren F. Screening for abdominal aortic aneurysm, a one-year follow up: an interview study. J Vasc Nurs 2010 Sep;28(3):97-101. PMID: 20709266. **KQ3E5.**

18. Biancari F, Mosorin M, Anttila V, et al. Ten-year outcome of patients with very small abdominal aortic aneurysm. Am J Surg 2002 Jan;183(1):53-5. PMID: 11869702. **KQ4E4a.**

19. Brady AR, Thompson SG, Greenhalgh RM, et al. Cardiovascular riskfactors and abdominal aortic aneurysm expansion: only smoking counts. Br J Surg 2003;90:492-3. PMID: None. **KQ2E10.**

20. Brady AR, Thompson SG, Fowkes FG, et al. Abdominal aortic aneurysm expansion: risk factors and time intervals for surveillance. Circulation 2004 Jul 6;110(1):16-21. PMID: 15210603. **KQ4E4a.**

21. Buckenham T, Roake J, Lewis D, et al. Abdominal aortic aneurysm surveillance: application of the UK Small Aneurysm Trial to a New Zealand tertiary hospital. N Z Med J 2007;120(1251):U2472. PMID: 17384700. **KQ2E5, KQ5E4.**

22. Collin J, Araujo L, Walton J, et al. Oxford screening programme for abdominal aortic aneurysm in men aged 65 to 74 years. Lancet 1988 Sep 10;2(8611):613-5. PMID: 2900988. **KQ1E4a.**

23. Collin J, Heather B, Walton J. Growth rates of subclinical abdominal aortic aneurysms-- implications for review and rescreening programmes. Eur J Vasc Surg 1991 Apr;5(2):141-4. PMID: 2037085. **KQ2E5.**

24. Conway AM, Malkawi AH, Hinchliffe RJ, et al. First-year results of a national abdominal aortic aneurysm screening programme in a single centre. Br J Surg 2012 Jan;99(1):73-7. PMID: 21928466. **KQ1E5.**

25. Cook TA, Galland RB. A prospective study to define the optimum rescreening interval for small abdominal aortic aneurysm. Cardiovasc Surg 1996 Aug;4(4):441-4. PMID: 8866077. **KQ2E10.**

26. Coughlin PA, Jackson D, White AD, et al. Meta-analysis of prospective trials determining the short- and mid-term effect of elective open and endovascular repair of abdominal aortic aneurysms on quality of life. Br J Surg 2012 Dec 19 PMID: 23254440. **KQ5E10.**

27. Couto E, Duffy SW, Ashton HA, et al. Probabilities of progression of aortic aneurysms: estimates and implications for screening policy. J Med Screen 2002;9(1):40-2. PMID: 11943797. **KQ2E5.**

28. Dangas G, O'Connor D, Firwana B, et al. Open versus endovascular stent graft repair of abdominal aortic aneurysms: a meta-analysis of randomized trials. Jacc: Cardiovascular Interventions 2012 Oct;5(10):1071-80. PMID: 23078738. **KQ5E10.**

29. Dawson JA, Choke E, Loftus IM, et al. A randomised placebo-controlled double-blind trial to evaluate lipid-lowering pharmacotherapy on proteolysis and inflammation in abdominal aortic aneurysms. Eur J Vasc Endovasc Surg 2011 Jan;41(1):28-35. PMID: 20880729. **KQ4E5.**

30. De Rango P, Cao P, Parlani G, et al. Outcome after endografting in small and large abdominal aortic aneurysms: a metanalysis. Eur J Vasc Endovasc Surg 2008 Feb;35(2):162-72. PMID: 18069023. **KQ4E9.**

31. De Rango P, Verzini F, Parlani G, et al. Quality of life in patients with small abdominal aortic aneurysm: the effect of early endovascular repair versus surveillance in the CAESAR trial. Eur J Vasc Endovasc Surg 2011 Mar;41(3):324-31. PMID: 21145269. **KQ4E5.**

32. Derubertis BG, Trocciola SM, Ryer EJ, et al. Abdominal aortic aneurysm in women: prevalence, risk factors, and implications for screening. J Vasc Surg 2007 Oct;46(4):630-5. PMID: 17903646. **KQ1E5.**

33. Dodd BR, Spence RA. Doxycycline inhibition of abdominal aortic aneurysm growth: a systematic review of the literature. Curr Vasc Pharmacol 2011 Jul 1;9(4):471-8. PMID: 21595625. **KQ4E8.**

34. Dubois L, Novick TV, Harris JR, et al. Outcomes after endovascular abdominal aortic aneurysm repair are equivalent between genders despite anatomic differences in women. Journal of Vascular Surgery 2013 Feb;57(2):382-9. PMID: 23266281. **KQ5E10.**

Appendix D. Excluded Studies

35. Duncan JL, Wolf B, Nichols DM, et al. Screening for abdominal aortic aneurysm in a geographically isolated area. Br J Surg 2005 Aug;92(8):984-8. PMID: 16034847. **KQ1E5.**

36. Duncan JL, Harrild KA, Iversen L, et al. Long term outcomes in men screened for abdominal aortic aneurysm: prospective cohort study. BMJ 2012;344:e2958. PMID: 22563092. **KQ2E4a.**

37. Dunne JA, Bailey MA, Griffin KJ, et al. Statins: The Holy Grail of Abdominal Aortic Aneurysm (AAA) Growth Attenuation? A Systematic Review of the Literature. Curr Vasc Pharmacol 2012 Jun 22 PMID: 22724473. **KQ3E8.**

38. Dynda DI, Andrews JA, Chiou AC, et al. Project PROMIS: Peoria Regional Outpatient Medical Imaging Study. Am J Surg 2008;195(3):322-7. PMID: 18308039. **KQ1E3.**

39. Fassiadis N, Roidl M, Stannett H, et al. Is screening of abdominal aortic aneurysm effective in a general practice setting? Int Angiol 2005 Jun;24(2):185-8. PMID: 15997221. **KQ1E5.**

40. Ferguson CD, Clancy P, Bourke B, et al. Association of statin prescription with small abdominal aortic aneurysm progression. Am Heart J 2010 Feb;159(2):307-13. PMID: 20152231. **KQ2E5.**

41. Filardo G, Powell JT, Martinez MA, et al. Surgery for small asymptomatic abdominal aortic aneurysms. [Review][Update of Cochrane Database Syst Rev. 2008;(4):CD001835; PMID: 18843626]. Cochrane Database of Systematic Reviews 2012;3:CD001835. PMID: 18843626. **KQ3E8.**

42. Fleming, C, Whitlock, E, Beil, T, et al. Primary care screening for abdominal aortic aneurysm. Evidence Synthesis Number 35. Rockville, MD: Agency for Healthcare Research and Quality; 2005. PMID: 20722131. **KQ1E8.**

43. Freiberg MS, Arnold AM, Newman AB, et al. Abdominal aortic aneurysms, increasing infrarenal aortic diameter, and risk of total mortality and incident cardiovascular disease events: 10-year follow-up data from the Cardiovascular Health Study. Circulation 2008 Feb 26;117(8):1010-7. PMID: 18268154. **KQ2E5.**

44. Gadowski GR, Pilcher DB, Ricci MA. Abdominal aortic aneurysm expansion rate: effect of size and beta-adrenergic blockade. J Vasc Surg 1994 Apr;19(4):727-31. PMID: 7909340. **KQ4E4a.**

45. Gibbs DM, Bown MJ, Hussey G, et al. The ectatic aorta: no benefit in surveillance. Annals of Vascular Surgery 2010 Oct;24(7):908-11. PMID: 20471205. **KQ2E7a.**

46. Golledge J, Muller R, Clancy P, et al. Evaluation of the diagnostic and prognostic value of plasma D-dimer for abdominal aortic aneurysm. Eur Heart J 2011 Feb;32(3):354-64. PMID: 20530504. **KQ2E5.**

47. Golledge J, Norman PE. Current status of medical management for abdominal aortic aneurysm. Atherosclerosis 2011 Jul;217(1):57-63. PMID: 21596379. **KQ4E8.**

48. Greco G, Egorova NN, Gelijns AC, et al. Development of a novel scoring tool for the identification of large >/=5 cm abdominal aortic aneurysms. Ann Surg 2010 Oct;252(4):675-82. PMID: 20881774. **KQ2E5.**

49. Grimshaw GM, Thompson JM, Hamer JD. Prevalence of abdominal aortic aneurysm associated with hypertension in an urban population. J Med Screen 1994 Oct;1(4):226-8. PMID: 8790525. **KQ1E5.**

50. Guessous I, Periard D, Lorenzetti D, et al. The efficacy of pharmacotherapy for decreasing the expansion rate of abdominal aortic aneurysms: a systematic review and meta-analysis. PLoS One 2008;3(3):e1895. PMID: 18365027. **KQ4E8.**

51. Hobbs S, Claridge M, Drage M, et al. Strategies to improve the effectiveness of abdominal aortic aneurysm screening programmes. J Med Screen 2004;11(2):93-6. PMID: 15153325. **KQ2E2.**

52. Huber TS, Wang JG, Derrow AE, et al. Experience in the United States with intact abdominal aortic aneurysm repair. J Vasc Surg 2001 Feb;33(2):304-10. PMID: 11174782. **KQ5E9.**

53. Hupp JA, Martin JD, Hansen LO. Results of a single center vascular screening and education program. J Vasc Surg 2007;46(2):182-7. PMID: 17664093. **KQ1E5.**

Appendix D. Excluded Studies

54. Jackson RS, Chang DC, Freischlag JA. Comparison of long-term survival after open vs endovascular repair of intact abdominal aortic aneurysm among Medicare beneficiaries. JAMA 2012 Apr 18;307(15):1621-8. PMID: 22511690. **KQ3E10, KQ5E10.**

55. Jamrozik K, Norman PE, Spencer CA, et al. Screening for abdominal aortic aneurysm: lessons from a population-based study. Med J Aust 2000 Oct 2;173(7):345-50. PMID: 11062788. **KQ1E5.**

56. Kanagasabay R, Gajraj H, Pointon L, et al. Co-morbidity in patients with abdominal aortic aneurysm. J Med Screen 1996;4(4):208-10. PMID: 9041487. **KQ1E5.**

57. Karlsson L, Bergqvist D, Lindback J, et al. Expansion of small-diameter abdominal aortic aneurysms is not reflected by the release of inflammatory mediators IL-6, MMP-9 and CRP in plasma. Eur J Vasc Endovasc Surg 2009 Apr;37(4):420-4. PMID: 19119028. **KQ4E5.**

58. Keeling WB, Armstrong PA, Stone PA, et al. An overview of matrix metalloproteinases in the pathogenesis and treatment of abdominal aortic aneurysms. Vasc Endovascular Surg 2005 Nov;39(6):457-64. PMID: 16382266. **KQ2E5.**

59. Kent KC, Zwolak RM, Egorova NN, et al. Analysis of risk factors for abdominal aortic aneurysm in a cohort of more than 3 million individuals. J Vasc Surg 2010 Sep;52(3):539-48. PMID: 20630687. **KQ2E5.**

60. Khaira HS, Herbert LM, Crowson MC. Screening for abdominal aortic aneurysms does not increase psychological morbidity. Ann R Coll Surg Engl 1998 Sep;80(5):341-2. PMID: 9849335. **KQ3E4a.**

61. Kim LG, Thompson SG, Marteau TM, et al. Screening for abdominal aortic aneurysms: the effects of age and social deprivation on screening uptake, prevalence and attendance at follow-up in the MASS trial. J Med Screen 2004;11(1):50-3. PMID: 15006116. **KQ1E5.**

62. Koning GG, Vallabhneni SR, Van Marrewijk CJ, et al. Procedure-related mortality of endovascular abdominal aortic aneurysm repair using revised reporting standards. Rev Bras Cir Cardiovasc 2007 Apr 13;22(1):7-13. PMID: 17992299. **KQ5E10.**

63. Koo V, Lau L, McKinley A, et al. Pilot study of sexual dysfunction following abdominal aortic aneurysm surgery. J Sex Med 2007 Jul;4(4:Pt 2):t-52. PMID: 17081220. **KQ5E10.**

64. Krohn CD, Kullmann G, Kvernebo K, et al. Ultrasonographic screening for abdominal aortic aneurysm. Eur J Surg 1992 Oct;158(10):527-30. PMID: 1360823. **KQ1E4a.**

65. Lall P, Gloviczki P, Agarwal G, et al. Comparison of EVAR and open repair in patients with small abdominal aortic aneurysms: can we predict results of the PIVOTAL trial? J Vasc Surg 2009 Jan;49(1):52-9. PMID: 19174250. **KQ4E4, KQ5E4.**

66. Laughlin GA, Allison MA, Jensky NE, et al. Abdominal aortic diameter and vascular atherosclerosis: the Multi-Ethnic Study of Atherosclerosis. Eur J Vasc Endovasc Surg 2011 Apr;41(4):481-7. PMID: 21236707. **KQ1E5.**

67. Laws C, Eastman J. Screening for abdominal aortic aneurysm by general practitioners and practice-based ultrasonographers. J Med Screen 2006;13(3):160-1. PMID: 17007659. **KQ1E5.**

68. Leach SD, Toole AL, Stern H, et al. Effect of beta-adrenergic blockade on the growth rate of abdominal aortic aneurysms. Arch Surg 1988 May;123(5):606-9. PMID: 2895995. **KQ4E4a.**

69. LeCroy CJ, Passman MA, Taylor SM, et al. Should endovascular repair be used for small abdominal aortic aneurysms? Vasc Endovascular Surg 2008;42(2):113-9. PMID: 18270271. **KQ5E4a.**

70. Lederle FA, Johnson GR, Wilson SE, et al. Prevalence and associations of abdominal aortic aneurysm detected through screening. Aneurysm Detection and Management (ADAM) Veterans Affairs Cooperative Study Group. Ann Intern Med 1997 Mar 15;126(6):441-9. PMID: 9072929. **KQ4E4a.**

71. Lederle FA, Johnson GR, Wilson SE, et al. The aneurysm detection and management study screening program: validation cohort and final results. Aneurysm Detection and Management Veterans Affairs Cooperative Study Investigators. Arch Intern Med 2000 May 22;160(10):1425-30. PMID: 10826454. **KQ4E4a.**

Appendix D. Excluded Studies

72. Lederle FA, Johnson GR, Wilson SE, et al. Quality of life, impotence, and activity level in a randomized trial of immediate repair versus surveillance of small abdominal aortic aneurysm. J Vasc Surg 2003 Oct;38(4):745-52. PMID: 14560224. **KQ4E5, KQ5E5.**

73. Lederle FA. Ultrasonographic screening for abdominal aortic aneurysms. Ann Intern Med 2003 Sep 16;139(6):516-22. PMID: 13679330. **KQ3E8.**

74. Lederle FA, Nelson DB, Joseph AM. Smokers' relative risk for aortic aneurysm compared with other smoking-related diseases: a systematic review. J Vasc Surg 2003 Aug;38(2):329-34. PMID: 12891116. **KQ1E5.**

75. Lee AJ, Fowkes FG, Carson MN, et al. Smoking, atherosclerosis and risk of abdominal aortic aneurysm. Eur Heart J 1997 Apr;18(4):671-6. PMID: 2009986. **KQ1E5.**

76. Lee ES, Pickett E, Hedayati N, et al. Implementation of an aortic screening program in clinical practice: implications for the Screen For Abdominal Aortic Aneurysms Very Efficiently (SAAAVE) Act. J Vasc Surg 2009 May;49(5):1107-11. PMID: 19307082. **KQ1E5.**

77. Leurs LJ, Buth J, Laheij RJ. Long-term results of endovascular abdominal aortic aneurysm treatment with the first generation of commercially available stent grafts. Arch Surg 2007 Jan;142(1):33v-41. PMID: 17224498. **KQ5E9.**

78. Lindeman JH, Abdul-Hussien H, Van Bockel JH, et al. Clinical trial of doxycycline for matrix metalloproteinase-9 inhibition in patients with an abdominal aneurysm: doxycycline selectively depletes aortic wall neutrophils and cytotoxic T cells. Circulation 2009 Apr 28;119(16):2209-16. PMID: 19364980. **KQ4E5.**

79. Lindholt JS, Henneberg EW, Fasting H, et al. Hospital based screening of 65-73 year old men for abdominal aortic aneurysms in the county of Viborg, Denmark. J Med Screen 1996;3(1):43-6. PMID: 8861051. **KQ1E5.**

80. Lindholt JS, Henneberg EW, Fasting H, et al. Mass or high-risk screening for abdominal aortic aneurysm. Br J Surg 1997 Jan;84(1):40-2. PMID: 9043447. **KQ1E5.**

81. Lindholt JS, Heegaard NH, Vammen S, et al. Smoking, but not lipids, lipoprotein(a) and antibodies against oxidised LDL, is correlated to the expansion of abdominal aortic aneurysms. Eur J Vasc Endovasc Surg 2001 Jan;21(1):51-6. PMID: 11170878. **KQ4E4a.**

82. Lindholt JS. Relatively high pulmonary and cardiovascular mortality rates in screening-detected aneurysmal patients without previous hospital admissions. Eur J Vasc Endovasc Surg 2007 Jan;33(1):94-9. PMID: 16893664. **KQ3E5.**

83. Lindholt JS, Norman P. Screening for abdominal aortic aneurysm reduces overall mortality in men. A meta-analysis of the mid- and long-term effects of screening for abdominal aortic aneurysms. Eur J Vasc Endovasc Surg 2008 Aug;36(2):167-71. PMID: 18485756. **KQ1E4.**

84. Lindholt JS, Sorensen HT, Michel JB, et al. Low-dose aspirin may prevent growth and later surgical repair of medium-sized abdominal aortic aneurysms. Vasc Endovascular Surg 2008 Aug;42(4):329-34. PMID: 18728038. **KQ4E4a.**

85. Lindholt JS, Norman PE. Meta-analysis of postoperative mortality after elective repair of abdominal aortic aneurysms detected by screening. Br J Surg 2011 May;98(5):619-22. PMID: 21374589. **KQ5E10.**

86. Lindsay SM, Duncan JL, Cairns J, et al. Geography, private costs and uptake of screening for abdominal aortic aneurysm in a remote rural area. BMC Public Health 2006;6:80. PMID: 16571121. **KQ1E5.**

87. MacSweeney ST, Ellis M, Worrell PC, et al. Smoking and growth rate of small abdominal aortic aneurysms. Lancet 1994 Sep 3;344(8923):651-2. PMID: 7915350. **KQ2E5.**

88. Mani K, Alund M, Bjorck M, et al. Screening for abdominal aortic aneurysm among patients referred to the vascular laboratory is cost-effective. Eur J Vasc Endovasc Surg 2010 Feb;39(2):208-16. PMID: 19942460. **KQ1E2.**

89. Marteau TM. Psychological costs of screening. BMJ 1989 Aug 26;299(6698):527. PMID: 2507059. **KQ3E4a.**

Appendix D. Excluded Studies

90. Marteau TM, Kim LG, Upton J, et al. Poorer self assessed health in a prospective study of men with screen detected abdominal aortic aneurysm: a predictor or a consequence of screening outcome? J Epidemiol Community Health 2004 Dec;58(12):1042-6. PMID: 15547070. **KQ3E5.**

91. Mastracci TM, Cina CS. Screening for abdominal aortic aneurysm in Canada: review and position statement of the Canadian Society for Vascular Surgery. J Vasc Surg 2007 Jun;45(6):1268-76. PMID: 17543696. **KQ1E8.**

92. McCollum P. Comments regarding 'Implications of attendance patterns in Northern Ireland for abdominal aortic aneurysm screening'. Eur J Vasc Endovasc Surg 2011 Oct;42(4):440-1. PMID: 21741281. **KQ1E4.**

93. Mell M, White JJ, Hill BB, et al. No increased mortality with early aortic aneurysm disease. Journal of Vascular Surgery 2012 Nov;56(5):1246-51. PMID: 22832264. **KQ1aE4a.**

94. Morris GE, Hubbard CS, Quick CR. An abdominal aortic aneurysm screening programme for all males over the age of 50 years. Eur J Vasc Surg 1994 Mar;8(2):156-60. PMID: 8181607. **KQ2E5.**

95. Mouawad NJ, Leichtle SW, Manchio JV, et al. Construct domain analysis of patient health-related quality of life: physical and mental trajectory profiles following open versus endovascular repair of abdominal aortic aneurysm. Patient Related Outcome Measures 2013;4:1-6. PMID: 23300352. **KQ5E10.**

96. Muehling BM, Halter G, Lang G, et al. Prospective randomized controlled trial to evaluate "fast-track" elective open infrarenal aneurysm repair. Langenbecks Arch Surg 2008 May;393(3):281-7. PMID: 18273636. **KQ4E9.**

97. Nicholls EA, Norman PE, Lawrence-Brown MM, et al. Screening for abdominal aortic aneurysms in Western Australia. Aust N Z J Surg 1992 Nov;62(11):858-61. PMID: 20169703. **KQ1E5.**

98. Norman PE, Jamrozik K, Lawrence BM, et al. Results of the Western Australian trial of screening for abdominal aortic aneurysms. ANZ J Surg 2005;75:A116. PMID: None. **KQ1E8.**

99. Norman PE, Jamrozik K, Lawrence-Brown MM, et al. Population based randomised controlled trial on impact of screening on mortality from abdominal aortic aneurysm. BMJ 2004 Nov 27;329(7477):1259. PMID: 15545293. **KQ1I1, KQ3I1.**

100. O'Kelly TJ, Heather BP. General practice-based population screening for abdominal aortic aneurysms: a pilot study. Br J Surg 1989 May;76(5):479-80. PMID: 2660948. **KQ1E4a.**

101. Ogren M, Bengtsson H, Bergqvist D, et al. Prognosis in elderly men with screening-detected abdominal aortic aneurysm. Eur J Vasc Endovasc Surg 1996 Jan;11(1):42-7. PMID: 8564486. **KQ1E4a.**

102. Ouriel K. Randomized clinical trials of endovascular repair versus surveillance for treatment of small abdominal aortic aneurysms. J Endovasc Ther 2009 Feb;16 Suppl 1:I94-105. PMID: 19317579. **KQ4E8.**

103. Padberg FT, Jr., Hauck K, Mercer RG, et al. Screening for abdominal aortic aneurysm with electronic clinical reminders. Am J Surg 2009 Nov;198(5):670-4. PMID: 19887197. **KQ1E5.**

104. PALOMBO D, LUCERTINI G, PANE B, et al. District-based abdominal aortic aneurysm screening in population aged 65 years and older. J Cardiovasc Surg 2010 Dec;51(6):777-82. PMID: 21124273. **KQ1E5.**

105. Patel MS, Brown DA, Wilson SE. Relevance of the ADAM and UK Small Aneurysm trial data in the age of endovascular aneurysm repair. Arch Surg 2009 Sep;144(9):806-10. PMID: 19797103. **KQ4E4a.**

106. Peach G, Holt P, Loftus I, et al. Questions remain about quality of life after abdominal aortic aneurysm repair. [Review]. Journal of Vascular Surgery 2012 Aug;56(2):520-7. PMID: 22840902. **KQ5E10.**

107. Powell JT. Long-term outcomes of immediate repair compared with surveillance of small abdominal aortic aneurysms. N Engl J Med 2002 May 9;346(19):1445-52. PMID: 12000814. **KQ5E5.**

108. Powell JT, Greenhalgh RM. Clinical practice. Small abdominal aortic aneurysms. N Engl J Med 2003 May 8;348(19):1895-901. PMID: 12736283. **KQ2E4.**

Appendix D. Excluded Studies

109. Prinssen M, Buskens E, Blankensteijn JD, et al. Quality of life endovascular and open AAA repair. Results of a randomised trial. Eur J Vasc Endovasc Surg 2004 Feb;27(2):121-7. PMID: 14718892. **KQ5E10.**

110. Raval MV, Eskandari MK. Outcomes of elective abdominal aortic aneurysm repair among the elderly: endovascular versus open repair. Surgery 2012 Feb;151(2):245-60. PMID: 21244863. **KQ5E10.**

111. Rothberg AD, McLeod H, Walters L, et al. Screening for abdominal aortic aneurysm--a pilot study in six medical schemes. S Afr Med J 2007 Jan;97(1):58-62. PMID: 17378284. **KQ1E5.**

112. Rughani G, Robertson L, Clarke M. Medical treatment for small abdominal aortic aneurysms. Cochrane Database Syst Rev 2012(9):CD009536. PMID: None. **KQ4E5, KQ5E5.**

113. Salem MK, Rayt HS, Hussey G, et al. Should Asian men be included in abdominal aortic aneurysm screening programmes? Eur J Vasc Endovasc Surg 2009 Dec;38(6):748-9. PMID: 19666232. **KQ1E5.**

114. Sampaio SM, Shin SH, Panneton JM, et al. Intraoperative endoleak during EVAR: frequency, nature, and significance. Vasc Endovascular Surg 2009 Aug;43(4):352-9. PMID: 19351648. **KQ5E9.**

115. Schermerhorn M, Zwolak R, Velazquez O, et al. Ultrasound screening for abdominal aortic aneurysm in medicare beneficiaries. Ann Vasc Surg 2008 Jan;22(1):16-24. PMID: 18055170. **KQ1E5.**

116. Schlosser FJ, Tangelder MJ, Verhagen HJ, et al. Growth predictors and prognosis of small abdominal aortic aneurysms. J Vasc Surg 2008 Jun;47(6):1127-33. PMID: 18440183. **KQ2E2, KQ5E5.**

117. Schlosser FJ, Vaartjes I, van der Heijden GJ, et al. Mortality after elective abdominal aortic aneurysm repair. Ann Surg 2010 Jan;251(1):158-64. PMID: 19838103. **KQ5E10.**

118. Schmidt T, Muhlberger N, Chemelli-Steingruber IE, et al. Benefit, risks and cost-effectiveness of screening for abdominal aortic aneurysm. Rofo 2010 Jul;182(7):573-80. PMID: 20563953. **KQ1E4.**

119. Schouten O, van Laanen JH, Boersma E, et al. Statins are associated with a reduced infrarenal abdominal aortic aneurysm growth. Eur J Vasc Endovasc Surg 2006 Jul;32(1):21-6. PMID: 16520071. **KQ4E4a.**

120. Scott RA, Kim LG, Ashton HA, et al. Assessment of the criteria for elective surgery in screen-detected abdominal aortic aneurysms. J Med Screen 2005;12(3):150-4. PMID: 16156946. **KQ2E5.**

121. Simoni G, Pastorino C, Perrone R, et al. Screening for abdominal aortic aneurysms and associated risk factors in a general population. Eur J Vasc Endovasc Surg 1995 Aug;10(2):207-10. PMID: 7655973. **KQ1E5.**

122. Simoni G, Gianotti A, Ardia A, et al. Screening study of abdominal aortic aneurysm in a general population: lipid parameters. Cardiovasc Surg 1996 Aug;4(4):445-8. PMID: 8866078. **KQ1E5.**

123. Singh K, Bonaa KH, Jacobsen BK, et al. Prevalence of and risk factors for abdominal aortic aneurysms in a population-based study : The Tromso Study. Am J Epidemiol 2001 Aug 1;154(3):236-44. PMID: 11479188. **KQ1E10.**

124. Smith FC, Grimshaw GM, Paterson IS, et al. Ultrasonographic screening for abdominal aortic aneurysm in an urban community. Br J Surg 1993 Nov;80(11):1406-9. PMID: 8252350. **KQ1E5.**

125. Spencer CA, Jamrozik K, Norman PE, et al. The potential for a selective screening strategy for abdominal aortic aneurysm. J Med Screen 2000;7(4):209-11. PMID: 11202589. **KQ1E5.**

126. Sukhija R, Aronow WS, Sandhu R, et al. Mortality and size of abdominal aortic aneurysm at long-term follow-up of patients not treated surgically and treated with and without statins. Am J Cardiol 2006 Jan 15;97(2):279-80. PMID: 16442379. **KQ4E4a.**

127. Svensjo S, Bjorck M, Gurtelschmid M, et al. Low prevalence of abdominal aortic aneurysm among 65-year-old Swedish men indicates a change in the epidemiology of the disease. Circulation 2011 Sep 6;124(10):1118-23. PMID: 21844079. **KQ1E5.**

128. Sweeting MJ, Thompson SG. Making predictions from complex longitudinal data, with application to planning monitoring intervals in a national screening programme. J R Stat Soc Ser A Stat Soc 2012 Apr;175(2):569-86. PMID: 22879705. **KQ2bE5.**

Appendix D. Excluded Studies

129. Takagi H, Matsui M, Umemoto T. A meta-analysis of clinical studies of statins for prevention of abdominal aortic aneurysm expansion. J Vasc Surg 2010 Dec;52(6):1675-81. PMID: 20638223. **KQ4E4a.**

130. Takagi H, Umemoto T. Reply to 'Comment on Effects of Statin Therapy on Abdominal Aortic Aneurysm Growth: A Meta-analysis and Meta-regression of Observational Comparative Studies'. European Journal of Vascular & Endovascular Surgery 2013 Jan;45(1):98-9. PMID: 23116985. **KQ3E4a.**

131. Takagi H, Goto SN, Matsui M, et al. A further meta-analysis of population-based screening for abdominal aortic aneurysm. J Vasc Surg 2010 Oct;52(4):1103-8. PMID: 20541347. **KQ1E8.**

132. Thomas SM, Beard JD, Ireland M, et al. Results from the prospective registry of endovascular treatment of abdominal aortic aneurysms (RETA): mid term results to five years. Eur J Vasc Endovasc Surg 2005 Jun;29(6):563-70. PMID: 15878530. **KQ5E10.**

133. Thompson AR, Cooper JA, Ashton HA, et al. Growth rates of small abdominal aortic aneurysms correlate with clinical events. Br J Surg 2010 Jan;97(1):37-44. PMID: 20013940. **KQ2E10.**

134. Twine CP, Williams IM. Systematic review and meta-analysis of the effects of statin therapy on abdominal aortic aneurysms. Br J Surg 2011 Mar;98(3):346-53. PMID: 21254006. **KQ4E4a.**

135. Twine CP, Williams IM. Authors' reply: Systematic review and meta-analysis of the effects of statin therapy on abdominal aortic aneurysms (Br J Surg 2011; 98: 362-353). Br J Surg 2011 May;98(5):745. PMID: 21462181. **KQ4E4a.**

136. United Kingdom Small Aneurysm Trial Participants. Smoking, lung function and the prognosis of abdominal aortic aneurysm. Eur J Vasc Endovasc Surg 2000 Jun;19(6):636-42. PMID: 10873733. **KQ4E5.**

137. van Lindert NH, Bienfait HP, Gratama JW, et al. Screening for aneurysm of the abdominal aorta: prevalence in patients with stroke or TIA. Eur J Neurol 2009 May;16(5):602-7. PMID: 19236464. **KQ1E3.**

138. Vardulaki KA, Prevost TC, Walker NM, et al. Growth rates and risk of rupture of abdominal aortic aneurysms. Br J Surg 1998 Dec;85(12):1674-80. PMID: 9876073. **KQ2E5.**

139. Vardulaki KA, Walker NM, Day NE, et al. Quantifying the risks of hypertension, age, sex and smoking in patients with aortic aneurysm. Br J Surg 2000 Feb;87(2):195-200. PMID: 10671927. **KQ1E5.**

140. Veroux P, D'Arrigo G, Veroux M, et al. Sexual dysfunction after elective endovascular or hand-assisted laparoscopic abdominal aneurysm repair. Eur J Vasc Endovasc Surg 2010 Jul;40(1):71-5. PMID: 20403714. **KQ5E4b.**

141. Vogel TR, Symons RG, Flum DR. Longitudinal outcomes after endovascular repair of abdominal aortic aneurysms. Vasc Endovascular Surg 2008 Oct;42(5):412-9. PMID: 18583307. **KQ5E10.**

142. Walton LJ, Franklin IJ, Bayston T, et al. Inhibition of prostaglandin E2 synthesis in abdominal aortic aneurysms: implications for smooth muscle cell viability, inflammatory processes, and the expansion of abdominal aortic aneurysms. Circulation 1999 Jul 6;100(1):48-54. PMID: 10393680. **KQ4E4a.**

143. Wang GJ, Carpenter JP. EVAR in small versus large aneurysms: does size influence outcome? Vasc Endovascular Surg 2009 Jun;43(3):244-51. PMID: 19088132. **KQ5E4a.**

144. Wanhainen A, Bergqvist D, Boman K, et al. Risk factors associated with abdominal aortic aneurysm: a population-based study with historical and current data. J Vasc Surg 2005 Mar;41(3):390-6. PMID: 15838468. **KQ1E5.**

145. Wilmink AB, Hubbard CS, Day NE, et al. Effect of propanolol on the expansion of abdominal aortic aneurysms: a randomized study. Br J Surg. 2000;87:499. **KQ4E4a.**

146. Wilmink AB, Hubbard CS, Day NE, et al. The incidence of small abdominal aortic aneurysms and the change in normal infrarenal aortic diameter: implications for screening. Eur J Vasc Endovasc Surg 2001 Feb;21(2):165-70. **KQ2E5.**

147. Wilmink AB, Vardulaki KA, Hubbard CS, et al. Are antihypertensive drugs associated with abdominal aortic aneurysms? J Vasc Surg 2002 Oct;36(4):751-7. PMID: 12368736. **KQ4E4a.**

Appendix D. Excluded Studies

148. Wilmink T, Claridge MW, Fries A, et al. A comparison between the short term and long term benefits of screening for abdominal aortic aneurysms from the Huntingdon Aneurysm screening programme. Eur J Vasc Endovasc Surg 2006 Jul;32(1):16-20. PMID: 16466938. **KQ1E4.**

149. Wilmink TB, Quick CR, Hubbard CS, et al. The influence of screening on the incidence of ruptured abdominal aortic aneurysms. J Vasc Surg 1999 Aug;30(2):203-8. PMID: 10436439. **KQ1E5, KQ2E5.**

150. Zarins CK, Crabtree T, Arko FR, et al. Endovascular repair or surveillance of patients with small AAA. Eur J Vasc Endovasc Surg 2005;29(5):496-503. PMID: 15966088. **KQ4E4, KQ5E4.**

151. Zarins CK, Crabtree T, Bloch DA, et al. Endovascular aneurysm repair at 5 years: Does aneurysm diameter predict outcome? J Vasc Surg 2006;44(5):920-9. **KQ4E4, KQ5E4.**

Appendix E Table 1. Methodological and Intervention Characteristics of Included One-time Screening Studies (KQs 1 and 3)

Characteristic	MASS[13,89,90]	Viborg[15,67,92-94]	Western Australian[16,95]	Chichester[14,25,91,124]	Wanhainen, 2004[104]	Lucarotti, 1997[105]
Study quality	Good	Good	Fair	Fair	Fair	Fair
N Randomized	67,800	12,639	41,000	15,775	NR	NR
Country	UK	Denmark	Australia	UK	Sweden	UK
Mean length of followup, y	13.1	13	3.6	15.0	1.0	1 month
Intervention	Ultrasound screening; patients with an aortic diameter of 3.0–4.4 cm were rescanned yearly. Those with an aortic diameter of 4.5–5.4 cm were rescanned at 3 month intervals. Urgent referral to a vascular surgeon was recommended for patients with aortic diameter ≥5.5 cm. QOL was assessed in patients with screen-detected AAA and those with normal scans at 1.5, 3, and 12 months.	Ultrasound screening; participants with aneurysms ≥5 cm were referred to a vascular surgeon; those with AAA 3–4.9 cm were offered annual scans to check for expansion. After 5 y those with initial ectatic aorta (diameter 2.5–2.9 cm) were offered rescreening. QOL (ScreenQL) was assessed 1 month after diagnosis, 1 month prior to annual screen, and 3–6 months after treatment.	Ultrasound screening*; QOL (SF-36, EuroQOL EQ-5D) was assessed 12 months after screening	Ultrasound screening; patients with an aneurysm of 3.0–4.4 cm diameter were rescanned annually and those with an aneurysm of 4.5–5.9 cm diameter were rescanned every 3 months. This was continued until February 1994 or until the patient died, underwent surgical intervention, or declined followup.	Participants were given a QOL assessment questionnaire (SF-36) at baseline and then 12 months after screening. A cohort of participants with screen-detected AAA were followed	Men invited to screening filled out the QOL questionnaire (General Health Questionnaire; linear analogue scale) prior to screening. 1 month after initial screening, the first 61 men with diagnosed AAA (definition NR) were asked to complete the QOL assessment again.
Control	Surveillance	Surveillance	Surveillance	Surveillance	Participants were given a QOL assessment questionnaire (SF-36) at baseline and 12 months after screening. A cohort of age-/sex-matched controls with normal AAA scans were followed.	Men invited to screening filled out the QOL questionnaire (General Health Questionnaire; linear analogue scale) prior to screening. 1 month after initial screening, the first 100 men with normal scans were asked to complete the QOL assessment again.
Benefit Outcomes Reported	1, 2, 3	1, 2, 3	1, 2, 3	1, 2, 3	1, 2, 3	NR

Appendix E Table 1. Methodological and Intervention Characteristics of Included One-time Screening Studies (KQs 1 and 3)

Characteristic	MASS[13,89,90]	Viborg[16,67,92-94]	Western Australian[16,95]	Chichester[14,25,91,124]	Wanhainen, 2004[104]	Lucarotti, 1997[105]
Harms Outcomes Reported	4, 5, 6	4, 5, 6	4, 5, 6	4, 5	6	6

Benefit outcomes: 1=all-cause mortality; 2=AAA-related mortality; 3=rupture (fatal and nonfatal).

Harm outcomes: 4=30-day operative mortality; 5=use of procedures (emergency and selective surgery); 6=quality of life.

*After screening, participants were given a letter containing the results of their scan and a copy for their primary care physician. Study staff made no further attempts to influence any aspect of clinical management after the scan was completed.

Abbreviations: AAA = abdominal aortic aneurysm; EQ-5D = EuroQOL-5D; MASS = Multicenter Aneurysm Screening Study; QOL = quality of life; SF-36 = Short-form 36-item Health Survey; NR = not reported.

Appendix E Table 2. Patient Characteristics of Included One-time Screening Studies (KQs 1 and 3)

Comparison	Study	Major inclusion criteria	Mean age % Female	% Current smoking	% Family history	% Diabetes	% CVD risk factors
Screening vs. no screening	MASS, 2002[13]	Men ages 65–74 y	69.2 0	NR	NR	NR	NR
	Chichester, 1995[14]	Patients ages 65–80 y	72* 59.0	NR	NR	NR	NR
	Viborg, 2005[15]	Men ages 64–73 y who lived in Viborg county	67.7 0	NR	NR	NR	NR
	Western Australian, 2004[16]	Men ages 65–79 y living in Perth and surrounding towns	72.6 0	NR	NR	NR	NR
Screening harms	Wanhainen, 2004[104]	Men and women ages 65–75 y with screen-detected AAA (≥3.0 cm) along with a group of those with a normal scan to act as controls	71 19.4	NR	NR	NR	NR
	Lucarotti, 1997[105]	Men born between 1925 and 1928 living in Gloucestershire and participating in the AAA screening program	NR 0	NR	NR	NR	NR

*Median.

Abbreviations: AAA = abdominal aortic aneurysm; MASS = Multicenter Aneurysm Screening Study; NR = not reported.

Appendix F Table 1. Percent of Screened Population With AAA of the Specified Size

Trial	Total Scanned	Total AAA (prevalence)	≥5.5 cm	5.0 to 5.9 cm	4.5 to 5.4 cm	3.0 to 4.4 cm
MASS, 2002[13]	27,147 (men)	1,333 (4.9)	166 (0.6)	NR	223 (0.8)	944 (3.5)
Chichester, 1995[14]	5,394 (men and women)	218 (4.0)	19 (0.4)	20 (0.4)	NR	179 (3.3)†
Western Australian, 2004[16]	12,213 (men)	875 (7.2)	61 (0.5)	NR	115 (0.9)	699 (5.7)
Viborg, 2005[15]	4,860 (men)	191 (3.9)	24 (0.5)	NR	NR	NR

*AAA >6.0 cm.
†AAA of 3.0 to 4.0 cm.

Abbreviations: AAA = abdominal aortic aneurysm; NR = not reported.

Appendix G Table 1. Methodological and Intervention Characteristics of Included Rescreening Studies (KQ 2)

Characteristic	D'Audiffret 2002[96]	Deveraj 2008[98]	Emerton 1994[102] McCarthy 2003[126] (5-y data) Crow 2001[103] (12-y data) Darwood 2012[17] (10-y data)	Hafez 2008[99]	Lederle 2000[101]	Lindholt 2000[100]	Scott 2001[97]
Study Quality	Fair	Fair	Fair	Fair	Good	Fair	Fair
N	223	999	50,130	22,961	15,098	6,339	1,011
N Analyzed	223	358	189 (5 y) 625 (5 y) 129 (12 y) 547 (10 y)	4,308	2,622	248	649
Country	US	UK	UK	UK	US	Denmark	UK
Mean length of followup, y	5.9	4	12	5*	4	5	10
Intervention	Patients from the ADAM trial; rescreening annually after aortic diameters of 2.5–2.9 cm were identified	Patients from the Good Hope Hospital Screening Program; rescreening of abnormal aortas (2.6–2.9 cm) at intervals ranging from 3 months to annually	Patients from the Gloucestershire Aneurysm Screening Study; rescreening at 5 and 12 y after a normal AAA scan	Patients from the Chichester Trial; rescreening at different intervals based on size of aorta at initial screening (2.5–2.9 cm: every 2 y (or once after 5 y); 3–4.4 cm annually; 4.5–5.4 cm every 3 months). Those with AAA ≥5.5 cm were sent to a surgical consultation with a vascular surgeon	Patients from the ADAM trial; rescreening in those found to have no AAA 4 y after initial screening	Case/control study of the Viborg Trial; annual followup screenings for AAA >3.0 cm and <3.0 cm; those with aorta 25–29 mm were offered rescreening 3 to 5 y after initial screen; control group were those with no AAA	Individuals with normal-sized aortas at initial scan were rescreened every 2 y. Patients with AAA 3–4.5 cm were scanned annually; 4.5–5.9 cm every 3 months. Patients were referred to a vascular surgeon once their aneurysm reached ≥6 cm. (These patients were NOT Chichester trial participants.)
Benefit outcomes reported	1, 2, 3	4	1, 2, 3, 4	2, 3, 4	1, 2	1†	2, 3, 4
Harm outcomes reported	6	NR	NR	5,6	NR	6	NR

Benefit outcomes: 1=all-cause mortality; 2=AAA-related mortality; 3=rupture (fatal and nonfatal); 4= AAA growth rate.
Harm outcomes: 5=30-day operative mortality; 6=use of procedures (emergency and selective surgery); 7=quality of life.
*Median.
†All-cause mortality reported, but not causes of death.

Abbreviations: AAA = abdominal aortic aneurysm; ADAM = Abdominal Aortic Aneurysm Detection and Management Study; NR = not reported.

Appendix G Table 2. Patient Characteristics of Included Rescreening Studies (KQ 2)

Study	Major inclusion criteria	Mean age % Female	% Current smoking	% Family history	% Diabetes	% CVD risk factors
D'Audiffret, 2002[96]	Those with aortic diameters of 2.5–2.9 cm	68.4 NR	81.6	13.9	11.2	PAD: 12.5 Hypertension: 49.8 Hypercholesterolemia: 17.5
Deveraj, 2008[98]	Men found to have ectatic aortas (2.6–2.9 cm in diameter) at first scan with a minimum of 1-y followup	74.8 0	NR	NR	NR	NR
Emerton, 1994[102] McCarthy 2003[126] (5-y data) Crow 2001[103] (12-y data) Darwood 2012[17] (10-y data)	Men ages 65–66 y at the time of original study who had aortic diameters <2.6 cm	NR 0	NR	NR	NR	NR
Hafez, 2008[99]	Men age 65 y invited to screen for AAA and found to have small AAA	65.6 0	NR	NR	NR	NR
Lederle, 2000[101]	VA patients ages 50–79 y without AAA (aortic diameters of ≤3.0 cm) who were part of the ADAM trial	66.6 2.4	No AAA: 14.6 AAA: 36.2	No AAA: 6.0 AAA: 2.7	No AAA: 17.6 AAA: 14.6	Hypertension: 55.2 High cholesterol: 41.9 CAD: 43.3 Any atherosclerosis: 50.5
Lindholt, 2000[100]	Men ages 65–73 y with either identified small AAA (2.5–2.9 cm) or those with a normal initial scan (along with 380 controls)	NR 0	NR	NR	NR	NR
Scott, 2001[97]	Male patients with a normal aorta on their initial scan at age 65 y	NR 0	NR	NR	NR	NR

Abbreviations: AAA = abdominal aortic aneurysm; CAD = coronary artery disease; CVD = cardiovascular disease; NR = not reported; PAD = peripheral artery disease; VA = Department of Veterans Affairs.

Appendix H Table 1. Methodological and Intervention Characteristics of Included Treatment Studies (KQs 4 and 5)

Study, Year	Study quality	N randomized	Country	Mean followup, y	Intervention	Control	Benefit outcomes reported	Harm outcomes reported
Open surgery vs. surveillance								
UKSAT, 1998[41,108,109,111,132]	Good	1,090	United Kingdom	4.6	Elective open surgery within 3 months of AAA identification	Surveillance until AAA reached 5.5 cm, rapidly increased in diameter (>1 cm/y) or developed symptoms	1, 2, 3	1, 2, 3
ADAM, 2002[106]	Good	1,136	United States	4.9	Elective open surgery within 6 weeks of AAA identification	Surveillance until AAA reached 5.5 cm, enlarged by at least 0.7 cm in 6 months/1.0 cm in 1 y, or symptoms developed	1, 2, 3	1, 2, 4
EVAR vs. surveillance								
CAESAR, 2010[113,114]	Fair	360	Italy	2.6‡	Patients received surgery via EVAR as soon as possible	Surveillance until AAA reached 5.5 cm in diameter, a rapid increase of >1 cm/y was found, or the aneurysm became symptomatic	1, 2, 3	2
PIVOTAL, 2010[115]	Fair	728	United States	1.7	Patients underwent EVAR ≤30 days of randomization	Surveillance until AAA reached 5.5 cm or enlarged ≥0.5 cm between any two 6-month assessments	1, 2, 3	1, 2
Pharmacotherapy vs. placebo								
Mosorin, 2001[118]	Fair	32	Finland	1.8	150 mg doxycycline daily	Placebo	1, 4	
Karlsson, 2009[119]	Fair	247	Sweden	1.5	600 mg azithromycin once daily for 3 days, followed by 600 mg once a week	Placebo	1, 2*, 4	2
Vammen, 2001[120]	Good	92	Denmark	2	300 mg oral roxithromycin once daily for 28 days	Placebo	1, 4†	2
PAT, 2002[116]	Good	552	Canada	2.5	20 mg propranolol twice a day; increased to 40 mg after 1 week, 80 mg after 2 weeks, and 120 mg at 4 weeks. Target dose was 80–120 mg twice a day	Placebo	1, 2, 3, 4	1, 2, 3
Lindholt, 1999[117]	Fair	54	Denmark	2	40 mg propranolol twice a day	Placebo	Not usable§	3
Registry studies								
Golledge, 2007[122]	Fair	NA	Australia	3.2‡	National audit examining the perioperative and intermediate results of EVAR for small AAA	NA	NA	1, 2, 5

Appendix H Table 1. Methodological and Intervention Characteristics of Included Treatment Studies (KQs 4 and 5)

Study, Year	Study quality	N randomized	Country	Mean followup, y	Intervention	Control	Benefit outcomes reported	Harm outcomes reported
Peppelenbosch, 2003[123]	Fair	NA	Europe	1.7	Audit of the EUROSTAR database of patients who had undergone elective EVAR for small AAA	NA	NA	1, 2, 5

Benefit outcomes: 1=all-cause mortality; 2=AAA-related mortality; 3=rupture (fatal and nonfatal); 4=AAA growth rate.

Harm outcomes: 1=30-day operative mortality; 2=use of procedures (emergency and selective surgery); 3=quality of life; 4=major complications associated with AAA open repair; 5=major complications associated with EVAR.

*No AAA-related death was found in both groups.

†This study also reported 5-y followup data on growth rate.

‡Median.

§Due to a large loss to followup, efficacy data were not usable. However, these losses were due to adverse events so the harms data are included.

Abbreviations: AAA = abdominal aortic aneurysm; ADAM = aAbdominal Aortic Aneurysm Detection and Management Study; CAESAR = Comparison of Surveillance vs. Aortic Endografting for Small Aneurysm Repair; N = sample size; NA = not applicable; EUROSTAR = European Collaborators on Stent-Graft Techniques for aAbdominal Aortic Aneurysm Repair; PAT = Propranolol Aneurysm Trial; PIVOTAL = Positive Impact of Endovascular Options for Treating Aneurysms Early; UKSAT = UK Small Aneurysm Trial.

Appendix H Table 2. Patient Characteristics of Included Treatment Studies (KQs 4 and 5)

Study	Major inclusion criteria	Mean age % Female	AAA diameter at baseline	% Current smoking	% Family history	% Diabetes	% CVD risk factors
Open surgery vs. surveillance							
UKSAT[108]	Patients ages 60–76 y with asymptomatic, small AAA (4.0–5.5 cm)	69.3 17.5	4.6	37.1	NR	2.5	Hypertension: 39 Probable ischemic heart disease: 14
ADAM[106]	Patients ages 50–79 y with AAA 4.0–5.4 cm identified via CT within the previous 12 weeks	68.1 0.8	4.7	39.2	12.9	9.8	Coronary disease: 41.9 Cerebrovascular disease: 12.4 Hypertension: 56.4
EVAR vs. surveillance							
CAESAR[113]	Patients ages 50–80 y; nonsymptomatic AAA 4.1–5.4 cm in diameter measured by CT within the previous 3 months	68.9 4.2	4.7	55.3	NR	13.6	Coronary disease: 39.2 Hypertension: 75.3
PIVOTAL[115]	Patients ages 40–90 y with AAA between 4.0 and 5.0 cm found by CT performed ≤3 months prior; eligible for EVAR	70.5 13.4	4.4	91.0	23.5	NR	MI: 31.3 CHF: 6.2 CAD: 55.4 PVD: 28.2 Hypertension: 77.8
Pharmacotherapy vs. surveillance							
Mosorin, 2001[118]	Aneurysm diameter perpendicular to the aortic axis of ≥3.0 cm in size or a ratio of infrarenal to suprarenal aortic diameter of ≥1.2 and a diameter <5.5 cm; followup of at least 6 months with 2 or more ultrasound examinations	68.4 9.4	3.3	35.4	NR	15.1	Hypertension: 40.2
Karlsson, 2009[119]	Patents age ≤80 y with AAA 3.5–4.9 cm	71† 18.5	NR	40	14	4.5	MI: 31.0 Stroke: 14.1 Hypertension: 62.5
Vammen, 2001[120]	AAA ≥3.0 cm detected by ultrasound the day of study entry; exclusively men	72.5 0	3.8	0.6‡	NR	NR	NR
PAT, 2002[116]	Asymptomatic small AAA (3.0–5.0 cm; some centers only, 3.0–4.5 cm) measured by ultrasound; no contraindications to study drug	68.9 16	3.8	34.7	NR	6.2	Angina: 14.8 Heart failure: 2.0 Claudication: 19.2 Hyperlipidemia: 33.6 Hypertension: 35.8 MI: 16.9 Stroke: 6.3
Lindholt, 1999[117]	Men with AAA 3.0–4.9 cm	69.2 0	3.4	NR	NR	NR	NR
Registry Studies							
Golledge, 2007[122]	Patients had to have undergone EVAR treatment for small AAA (≤5.5 cm)	75† 16	NR	11	NR	11	Hypertension: 67 Ischemic heart disease*: 54 CVD: 5 PVD: 26

Appendix H Table 2. Patient Characteristics of Included Treatment Studies (KQs 4 and 5)

Study	Major inclusion criteria	Mean age % Female	AAA diameter at baseline	% Current smoking	% Family history	% Diabetes	% CVD risk factors
Peppelenbosch, 2003[123]	Patients in the EUROSTAR database who had undergone elective EVAR to repair an AAA; minimal followup of 1 month; vascular anatomy suitable for implantation of a stent graft	69.7 7	NR	NR	NR	NR	History of cardiac symptoms: 56

*Defined as angina, MI, arrhythmia, or heart failure.
†Median.
‡Mean.

Abbreviations: AAA = abdominal aortic aneurysm; ADAM = Abdominal Aortic Aneurysm Detection and Management Study; CAD = coronary artery disease; CAESAR = Comparison of Surveillance Versus Aortic Endografting for Small Aneurysm Repair; CHF = congestive heart failure; CT = computed tomography; CVD = cardiovascular disease; EUROSTAR = European Collaborators on Stent-Graft Techniques for Abdominal Aortic Aneurysm Repair; EVAR = endovascular aneurysm repair; MI = myocardial infarction; NR = not reported; PAT = Propranolol Aneurysm Trial; PIVOTAL = Positive Impact of Endovascular Options for Treating Aneurysms Early; PVD = peripheral vascular disease; UKSAT = UK Small Aneurysm Trial.

Appendix I Table 1. Quality of Life Results in Studies of Treatment for Small AAA (KQs 4 and 5)

Study	QOL screening method	Time period	Treatment Group	N Analyzed	QOL scores, mean (SD)¶	Mean difference (95% CI), p-value
Open surgery vs. surveillance						
UKSAT[132]	MOS subscale*	Baseline	IG	480	Physical function: 64.2 (30.7) Mental health: 80.2 (17.2)	Physical function: -2.3 (-6.0 to 1.5); NR Mental health: 0.7 (-1.5 to 2.8); NR
			CG	512	Physical function: 66.5 (29.3) Mental health: 79.5 (17.0)	
		12 months post-randomization	IG	429	Physical function: 62.1 (29.9) Mental health: 81.7 (17.9) *Mean difference from BL:* Physical function: -3.5 (-6.1 to -0.8) Mental health: 0 (-1.5 to 1.5)	Physical function: 1.7 (-2.3 to 5.7) Mental health: 2.1 (-0.4 to 4.5)
			CG	436	Physical function: 60.3 (30.2) Mental health: 79.6 (18.6) *Mean difference from BL:* Physical function: -6.2 (-8.8 to -3.7) Mental health: 0 (1.7 to 1.8)	
EVAR vs. surveillance						
CAESAR[114]	SF-36*	Baseline through 6 months post-randomization	IG	173	*Mean difference (95% CI) from BL:* Overall QOL: 4.6 (2.3 to 7) Physical functioning: -0.6 (-3.7 to 2.4) Mental health: 5.2 (2.8 to 7.5)	*IG vs. CG* Overall QOL: 5.4 (2.1 to 8.8); p=0.002 Physical function: 3.8 (0.5 to 7.2); p=0.02 Mental health: 6.0 (2.7 to 9.3); p=0.0005
			CG	166	*Mean difference (95% CI) from BL:* Overall QOL: -0.8 (-3.2 to 1.6) Physical functioning: -4.3 (-7.3 to -1.2) Mental health: -0.8 (-3.2 to 1.5)	
		Baseline through end of followup§	IG	173	*Mean difference (95% CI) from BL:* Overall QOL: 4.6 (2.3 to 7) Physical functioning: -0.6 (-3.7 to 2.4) Mental health: 5.2 (2.8 to 7.5)	*IG vs. CG* Overall QOL: 2.4 (-1.7 to 6.6); p=0.25 Physical function: 1.5 (-2.6 to 5.5); p=0.48 Mental health: 2.0 (-2.4 to 6.4); p=0.38
			CG	166	*Mean difference (95% CI) from BL:* Overall QOL: -6.3 (-9.3 to -3.4)‖ Physical functioning: -8.2 (-12.0 to -4.4) Mental health: 4.8 (-7.9 to -1.7)‖	
Pharmacotherapy vs. surveillance						
Lindholt 1999[117]	ScreenQL*†	Baseline through 2 y	IG	30	NR	Overall QOL: -5.83 (6.2)‡; p=0.05 Emotional domain: -0.35 (2.1)‡; p=0.59 Health perception: -1.39 (2.98)‡; p=0.13
			CG	24	NR	Overall QOL: -1.70 (5.5)‡; p=0.07 Emotional domain: 0.00 (2.0)‡; p=0.69 Health perception: -0.38 (2.10)‡; p=0.30

Appendix I Table 1. Quality of Life Results in Studies of Treatment for Small AAA (KQs 4 and 5)

Study	QOL screening method	Time period	Treatment Group	N Analyzed	QOL scores, mean (SD)¶	Mean difference (95% CI), p-value
PAT 2002[116]	SF-36*	Baseline	IG	276	Physical function: 70.8 (23.9) Mental health: 78.9 (17.3)	Physical function: p=0.11 Mental health: p=0.45
			CG	272	Physical function: 74.1 (24.0) Mental health: 77.8 (17.9)	
		1 month post-randomization	IG	276	Physical function: 68.9 (18.9) Mental health: 78.9 (17.6)	Physical function: p=0.006 Mental health: p=0.58
			CG	272	Physical function: 74.4 (23.8) Mental health: 78.3 (17.5)	

*Lower score denotes poorer status.
†A validated generic and global QOL questionnaire with 24 items evaluating 6 categories: general QOL, emotional health, physical health, psychosomatic distress, social and family functions, and marriage.
‡Mean (SD); change from BL in each group, not IG vs. CG.
§Mean, 3 y from BL (SD, 1.2 y).
‖ p<0.01.
¶Only summary scores reported here. For complete subscales please see full text.

Abbreviations: BL = baseline; CAESAR = Comparison of Surveillance Versus Aortic Endografting for Small Aneurysm Repair; CG = control group; EVAR = endovascular aneurysm repair; IG = intervention group; MOS = Medical Outcomes Study; NR = not reported; PAT = Propanolol Aneurysm Trial; QOL = quality of life; SF-36 = Short-Form 36-Item Health Survey; UKSAT = UK Small Aneurysm Trial.

Appendix J. AAA Clinical Recommendations From Expert Groups

Expert Group	Target Group	Starting Age	Stopping Age	Frequency of Screening	Surveillance	Intervention(s)	Recommendation Grade
USPSTF, 2005[1]	Men who have ever smoked	65	75	One time	NR	EVAR or OSR if AAA ≥5.5 cm	B Recommendation *The service is recommended.*
ACC, 2005[168]	Men who are siblings or offspring of patients with AAA	≥60	75	One time	Every 6–12 months if AAA 4.0–5.4 cm; every 2–3 y if AAA smaller than 4.0 cm	Elective open repair if AAA ≥5.5 cm and low- or average-risk patient; endograft repair if AAA ≥5.5 cm and high-risk patient	Class I *Recommendation that procedure or treatment is useful/effective.* Level of Evidence: B *Evidence from single RCT or nonrandomized studies.*
ACC, 2005[168]	Men ages 65–75 y who ever smoked	65	75	One time	Every 6–12 months if AAA 4.0–5.4 cm; every 2–3 y if AAA smaller than 4.0 cm.	Elective open repair if AAA ≥5.5 cm and low- or average-risk patient; endograft repair if AAA ≥5.5 cm and high-risk patient.	Class IIA *Recommendation in favor of treatment or procedure being useful/effective.* Level of Evidence: B *Some conflicting evidence from single RCT or nonrandomized studies.*
CSVS, 2007[167]	Men	65	75	Every 3–5 y	Policy is unclear for AAA 4.4–5.4 cm; annually if AAA 3.0–4.4 cm	Surgical repair (not specified) if AAA ≥5.5 cm	Grade 1A *Evidence obtained from at least 1 properly randomized controlled trial or 1 large epidemiological study. Evidence sufficient for universal use.*
CSVS, 2007[167]	Women age 65 y or older with multiple risk factors (smoking history, CVD, family history of AAA)	65	NR	Every 3–5 y	Policy is unclear for AAA 4.4–5.4 cm; annual rescreening if AAA 3.0–4.4 cm	Surgical repair (not specified) if AAA ≥5.5 cm	Grade 3C *Opinions of respective authorities, based on clinical experience, descriptive studies, or reports of expert committees. Evidence not based on RCTs.*
CSVS, 2007[167]	Women age 65 y or older, all adults age <65 y, and men age 75–80 y	NA	NA	NA	NA	NA	Grade 3C *Opinions of respective authorities, based on clinical experience, descriptive studies, or reports of expert committees. Evidence not based on RCTs.*
CCS, 2005[169]	Men ages 65–74 y	NR	NR	Every 3–5 y	Repeat ultrasound every 6 months if AAA ≥4.5 cm, repeat in 1 y if AAA 4.0–4.5 cm; repeat in 2 y if AAA 3.5–3.9 cm; repeat in 3 y if AAA 3.1–3.4 cm	Referral to vascular surgeon if AAA ≥4.5 cm; surgical repair (not specified) if AAA >5.5 cm in men and >4.5 in women. Consider surgical repair if growth >1 cm in 1 y	Grade 1A *Evidence obtained from at least 1 properly randomized controlled trial or 1 large epidemiological study. Evidence sufficient for universal use.*

Appendix J. AAA Clinical Recommendations From Expert Groups

Expert Group	Target Group	Starting Age	Stopping Age	Frequency of Screening	Surveillance	Intervention(s)	Recommendation Grade
CCS, 2005[169]	Women age 65 y or older with CVD and positive family history of AAA	65	NR	Every 3–5 y	Repeat ultrasound every 6 months if AAA ≥4.5 cm; repeat in 1 y if AAA 4.0–4.5 cm; repeat in 2 y if AAA 3.5–3.9 cm; repeat in 3 y if AAA 3.1–3.4 cm	Referral to vascular surgeon if AAA ≥4.5 cm; surgical repair (not specified) if AAA >5.5 cm in men and >4.5 cm in women. Consider surgical repair if growth >1 cm in 1 y	Grade 3C *Opinions of respective authorities, based on clinical experience, descriptive studies, or reports of expert committees. Evidence not based on RCTs.*
SVS, 2009[24]	Men age 50 y or older and family history of AAA	50	64	One time	Every 6 months if AAA 4.5–5.4 cm; at 1 y if AAA 3.5–4.4 cm; repeat in 3 y if AAA 3.0–3.4 cm; repeat in 5 y if AAA 2.6–2.9 cm	Surgical repair if fusiform AAA ≥5.5 cm, secular AAA, young healthy patients and especially women with AAA 5.0–5.4 cm, statins, smoking cessation, ACE inhibitors/angiotensin receptor blockers; EVAR is associated with lower risk than OSR	Grade 3C *Opinions of respective authorities, based on clinical experience, descriptive studies, or reports of expert committees. Evidence not based on RCTs.*
SVS, 2009[24]	Men age 65 y or older; as early as 55 years for those with a family history of AAA	65 (55 if family history of AAA)	NR	One time	Repeat every 6 months if AAA 4.0–4.5 cm; annual examination if AAA 3.0–4.0 cm	Refer to a vascular specialist if AAA >4.5 cm; surgical repair if >5.5 cm; EVAR is associated with lower risk than OSR	Level of recommendation: Strong *Benefits > Risks* Quality of evidence: High *Additional research is considered very unlikely to change confidence in the estimate of effect.*
SVS, 2009[24]	Women age 65 y or older with a family history of AAA or who have smoked	65	NR	One time	Repeat every 6 months if AAA 4.0–4.5 cm; annual examination if AAA 3.0–4.0 cm	Refer to a vascular specialist if AAA >4.5 cm; surgical repair if >5.5 cm; EVAR is associated with lower risk than OSR	Level of recommendation: Strong *Benefits > Risks* Quality of evidence: Moderate *Further research is likely to have an important impact on in the estimate of effect.*

Abbreviations: AAA = abdominal aortic aneurysm; ACC = American College of Cardiology; ACE = angiotensin-converting enzyme; CCS = Canadian Cardiovascular Society; CSVS = Canadian Society for Vascular Surgery; CVD = cardiovascular disease; EVAR = endovascular aneurysm repair; NR = not reported; OSR = open surgical repair; RCT = randomized, controlled trial; SVS = Society of Vascular Surgery; USPSTF = U.S. Preventive Services Task Force.

Appendix K Figure 1. Sensitivity Analysis of AAA-Related Mortality in One-Time Screening Trials (KQ 1)

Study	Year	Men (%)	Mean follow-up (years)		HR (95% CI)	% Weight
Follow up at 3-5 years						
MASS	2002	100%	4.1		0.58 (0.42, 0.78)	68.80
Viborg	2005	100%	4.3		0.33 (0.16, 0.71)	31.20
Subtotal (I-squared = 46.7%, p = 0.171)					0.49 (0.29, 0.81)	100.00
Follow up at 6-7 years						
MASS	2007	100%	7		0.53 (0.42, 0.68)	100.00
Subtotal (I-squared = .%, p = .)					0.53 (0.42, 0.67)	100.00
Follow up at 10-11 years						
MASS	2009	100%	10.1		0.52 (0.43, 0.63)	59.51
Viborg	2006	100%	9.6		0.27 (0.15, 0.49)	40.49
Subtotal (I-squared = 76.6%, p = 0.039)					0.40 (0.21, 0.75)	100.00
Follow up at 13-15 years						
Chichester	2007	100%	15		0.89 (0.60, 1.32)	32.03
MASS	2012	100%	13.1		0.58 (0.49, 0.69)	41.68
Viborg	2010	100%	13		0.34 (0.20, 0.57)	26.29
Subtotal (I-squared = 76.4%, p = 0.014)					0.58 (0.38, 0.88)	100.00

NOTE: Weights are from random effects analysis

```
          .8  1 1.2
Favors screening    Favors no screening
```

Appendix K Figure 2. Pooled Analysis of AAA-Related Mortality in One-Time Screening Trials (Peto Odds Ratio)

Study	Year	Men (%)	Mean follow-up (years)		Odds ratio (95% CI)	Events, Treatment	Events, Control	% Weight
Follow up at 3-5 years								
Chichester	1995	100%	5		0.60 (0.28, 1.27)	10/3205	17/3228	9.49
MASS	2002	100%	4.1		0.58 (0.44, 0.78)	65/33839	113/33961	62.67
Viborg	2005	100%	4.3		0.37 (0.19, 0.70)	9/6333	27/6306	12.67
W. Australian	2004	100%	3.6		0.72 (0.40, 1.31)	18/19352	25/19352	15.16
Subtotal (I-squared = 0.0%, p = 0.490)					0.57 (0.45, 0.72)	102/62729	182/62847	100.00
Follow up at 6-7 years								
MASS	2007	100%	7		0.54 (0.43, 0.68)	105/33883	196/33887	86.24
Viborg	2007	100%	5.9		0.28 (0.16, 0.50)	9/6333	39/6306	13.76
Subtotal (I-squared = 77.2%, p = 0.036)					0.50 (0.40, 0.61)	114/40216	235/40193	100.00
Follow up at 10-11 years								
Chichester	2002	100%	10		0.79 (0.46, 1.34)	24/3000	31/3058	9.61
MASS	2009	100%	10.1		0.53 (0.44, 0.64)	155/33883	296/33887	78.99
Viborg	2006	100%	9.6		0.32 (0.19, 0.52)	14/6333	51/6303	11.40
Subtotal (I-squared = 68.7%, p = 0.041)					0.52 (0.44, 0.61)	193/43216	378/43248	100.00
Follow up at 13-15 years								
Chichester	2007	100%	15		0.88 (0.60, 1.31)	47/2995	54/3045	12.86
MASS	2012	100%	13.1		0.59 (0.50, 0.70)	224/33883	381/33887	77.62
Viborg	2010	100%	13		0.37 (0.24, 0.59)	19/6333	55/6303	9.52
Subtotal (I-squared = 74.5%, p = 0.020)					0.60 (0.52, 0.69)	290/43211	490/43235	100.00

.8 1 1.2

Favors screening   Favors no screening

Appendix K Figure 3. Pooled Analysis of AAA-Related Mortality in One-Time Screening Trials (Outcome Data Pooled at the Longest Followup)

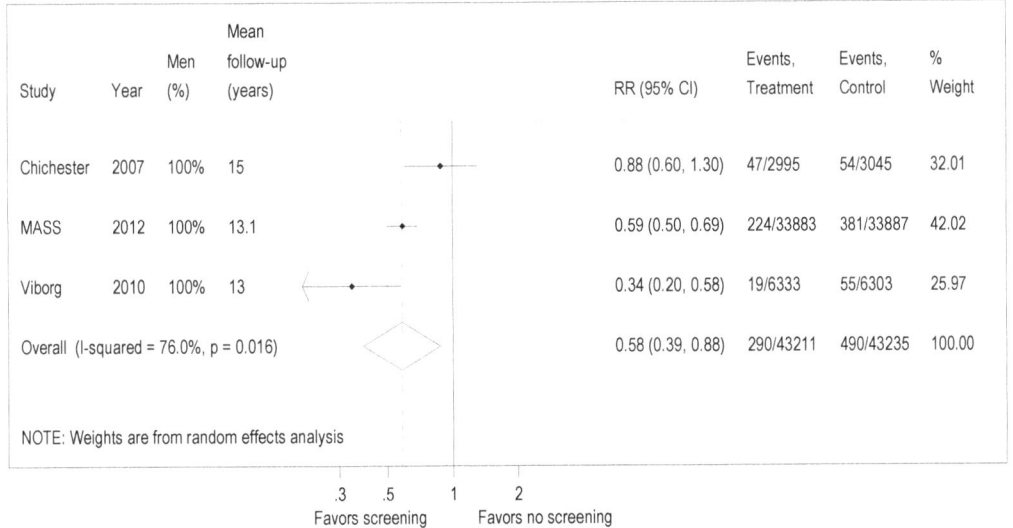

Study	Year	Men (%)	Mean follow-up (years)	RR (95% CI)	Events, Treatment	Events, Control	% Weight
Chichester	2007	100%	15	0.88 (0.60, 1.30)	47/2995	54/3045	32.01
MASS	2012	100%	13.1	0.59 (0.50, 0.69)	224/33883	381/33887	42.02
Viborg	2010	100%	13	0.34 (0.20, 0.58)	19/6333	55/6303	25.97
Overall (I-squared = 76.0%, p = 0.016)				0.58 (0.39, 0.88)	290/43211	490/43235	100.00

NOTE: Weights are from random effects analysis

.3 .5 1 2
Favors screening   Favors no screening

Appendix K Figure 4. Funnel Plot of AAA-Related Mortality at 3 to 5 Years in One-Time Screening Trials (KQ 1)

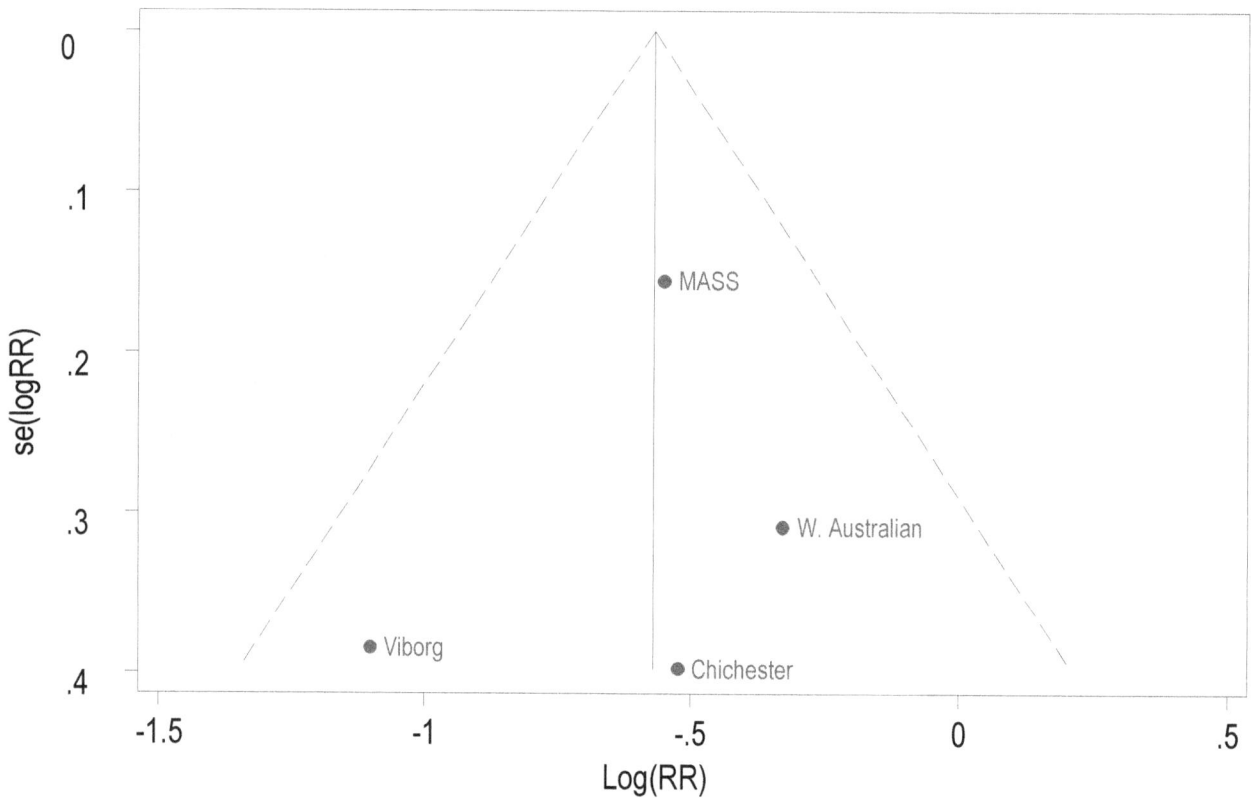

Appendix K Figure 5. Sensitivity Analyses of All-Cause Mortality in One-Time Screening Trials (KQ 1)

Study	Year	Men (%)	Mean follow-up (years)		HR (95% CI)	% Weight
Follow up at 3-5 years						
MASS	2002	100%	4.1		0.97 (0.93, 1.02)	75.40
Viborg	2005	100%	4.3		0.92 (0.84, 1.00)	24.60
Subtotal (I-squared = 9.5%, p = 0.293)					0.96 (0.92, 1.00)	100.00
Follow up at 6-7 years						
MASS	2007	100%	7		0.96 (0.93, 1.00)	100.00
Subtotal (I-squared = .%, p = .)					0.96 (0.93, 1.00)	100.00
Follow up at 10-11 years						
MASS	2009	100%	10.1		0.97 (0.95, 1.00)	85.36
Viborg	2006	100%	9.6		0.97 (0.91, 1.03)	14.64
Subtotal (I-squared = 0.0%, p = 1.000)					0.97 (0.95, 0.99)	100.00
Follow up at 13-15 years						
Chichester	2007	100%	15		1.01 (0.95, 1.07)	9.37
MASS	2012	100%	13.1		0.97 (0.95, 0.99)	77.92
Viborg	2010	100%	13		0.98 (0.93, 1.03)	12.71
Subtotal (I-squared = 0.0%, p = 0.443)					0.97 (0.96, 0.99)	100.00

NOTE: Weights are from fixed effects analysis

.8   1   1.2

Favors screening   Favors no screening

Appendix K Figure 6. Pooled Analysis of All-Cause Mortality in One-Time Screening Trials (Outcome Data Pooled at Longest Followup)

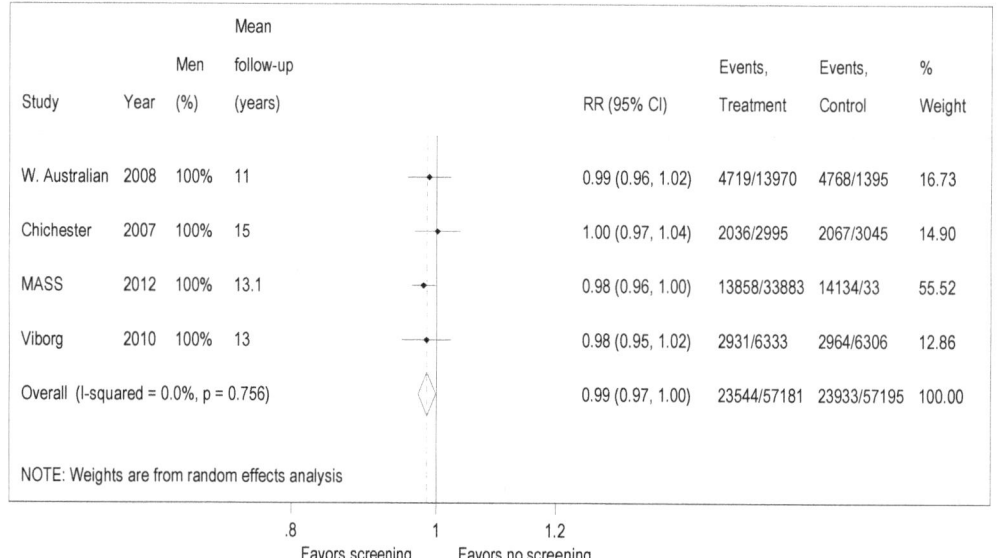

Study	Year	Men (%)	Mean follow-up (years)	RR (95% CI)	Events, Treatment	Events, Control	% Weight
W. Australian	2008	100%	11	0.99 (0.96, 1.02)	4719/13970	4768/1395	16.73
Chichester	2007	100%	15	1.00 (0.97, 1.04)	2036/2995	2067/3045	14.90
MASS	2012	100%	13.1	0.98 (0.96, 1.00)	13858/33883	14134/33	55.52
Viborg	2010	100%	13	0.98 (0.95, 1.02)	2931/6333	2964/6306	12.86
Overall (I-squared = 0.0%, p = 0.756)				0.99 (0.97, 1.00)	23544/57181	23933/57195	100.00

NOTE: Weights are from random effects analysis

.8   1   1.2

Favors screening   Favors no screening

Appendix K Figure 7. Funnel Plot of All-Cause Mortality at 3 to 5 Years in One-Time Screening Trials (KQ 1)

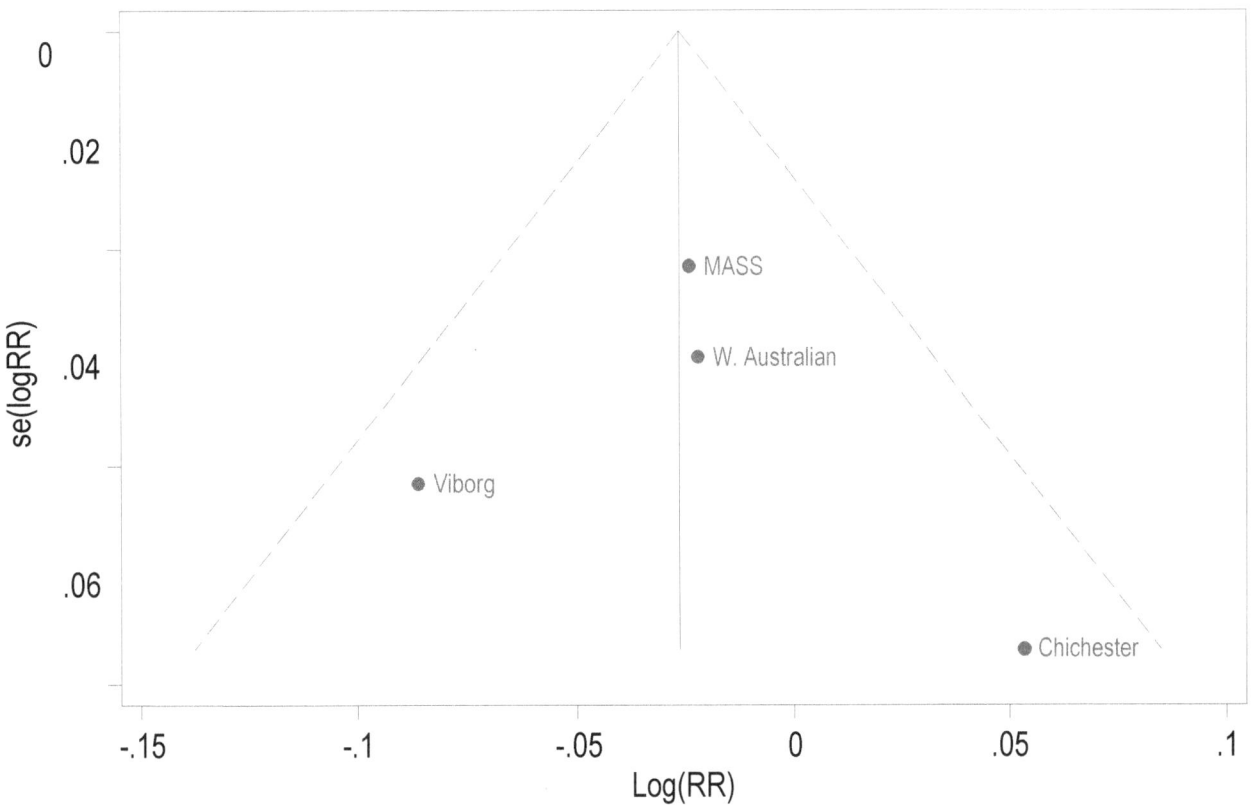

Appendix K Figure 8. Sensitivity Analyses of AAA Rupture in One-Time Screening Trials (KQ 1): Hazard Ratios

Study	Year	Men (%)	Mean follow-up (years)		HR (95% CI)	% Weight
Follow up at 3-5 years						
Viborg	2005	100%	4.3		0.27 (0.13, 0.60)	100.00
Subtotal (I-squared = .%, p = .)					0.27 (0.13, 0.58)	100.00
Follow up at 6-7 years						
MASS	2007	100%	7		0.52 (0.42, 0.64)	100.00
Subtotal (I-squared = .%, p = .)					0.52 (0.42, 0.64)	100.00
Follow up at 13-15 years						
Chichester	2007	100%	15		0.88 (0.61, 1.26)	42.45
MASS	2012	100%	13.1		0.57 (0.49, 0.66)	57.55
Subtotal (I-squared = 78.8%, p = 0.030)					0.69 (0.45, 1.04)	100.00

NOTE: Weights are from random effects analysis

.8 1 1.2

Favors screening   Favors no screening

Appendix K Figure 9. Pooled Analysis of AAA Rupture in One-Time Screening Trials (Outcome Data Pooled at the Longest Followup)

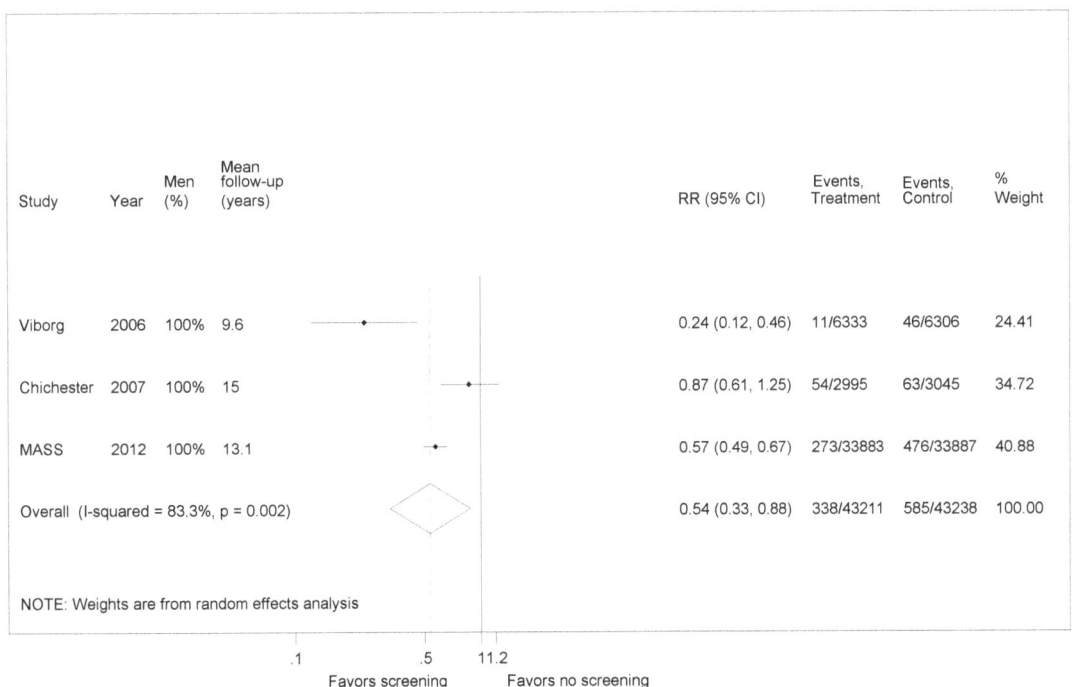

Study	Year	Men (%)	Mean follow-up (years)	RR (95% CI)	Events, Treatment	Events, Control	% Weight
Viborg	2006	100%	9.6	0.24 (0.12, 0.46)	11/6333	46/6306	24.41
Chichester	2007	100%	15	0.87 (0.61, 1.25)	54/2995	63/3045	34.72
MASS	2012	100%	13.1	0.57 (0.49, 0.67)	273/33883	476/33887	40.88
Overall (I-squared = 83.3%, p = 0.002)				0.54 (0.33, 0.88)	338/43211	585/43238	100.00

NOTE: Weights are from random effects analysis

Favors screening   Favors no screening

Appendix K Figure 10. Funnel Plot of AAA Rupture at 3 to 5 Years in One-Time Screening Trials (KQ 1)

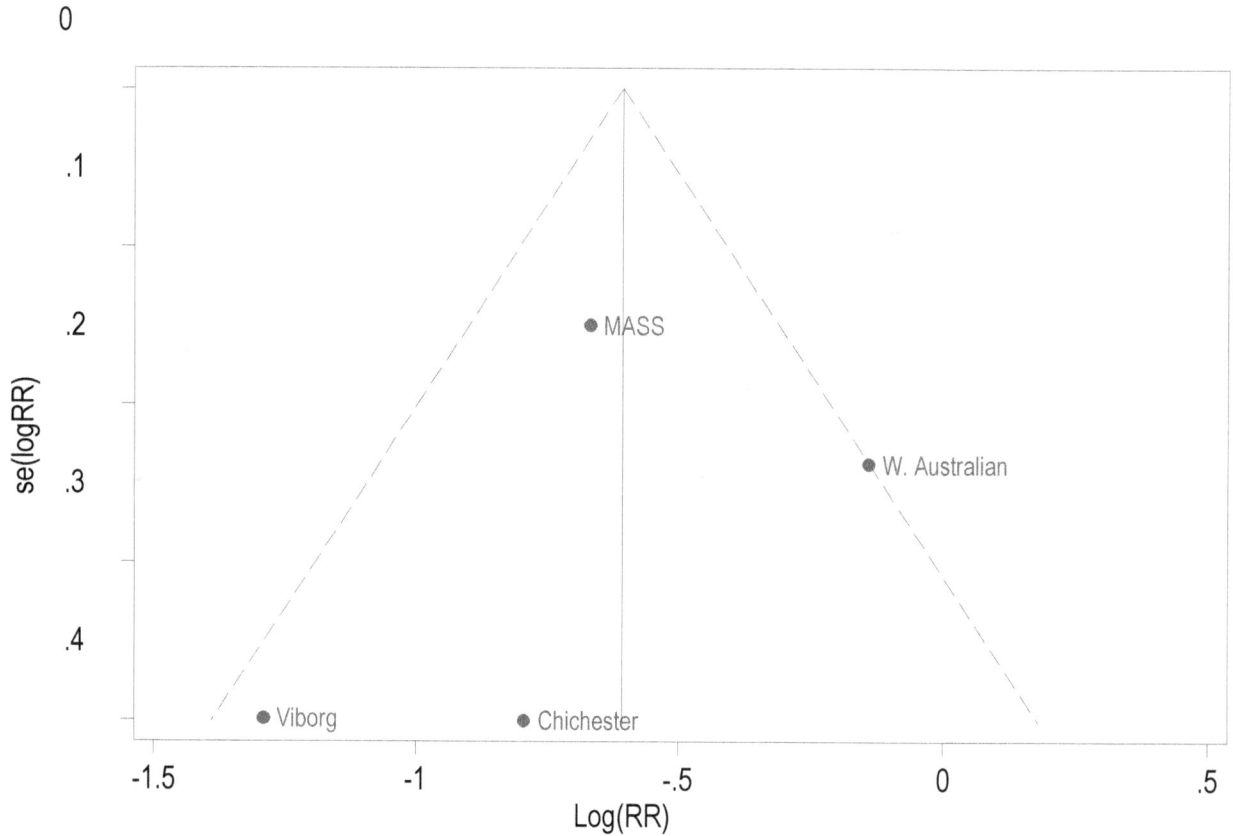

Appendix K Figure 11. Pooled Analysis of All-Cause Mortality, AAA-Related Mortality, and Rupture in Open Surgery vs. Surveillance Trials at 5-Year Followup (Fixed-Effects Model) (KQ 4)

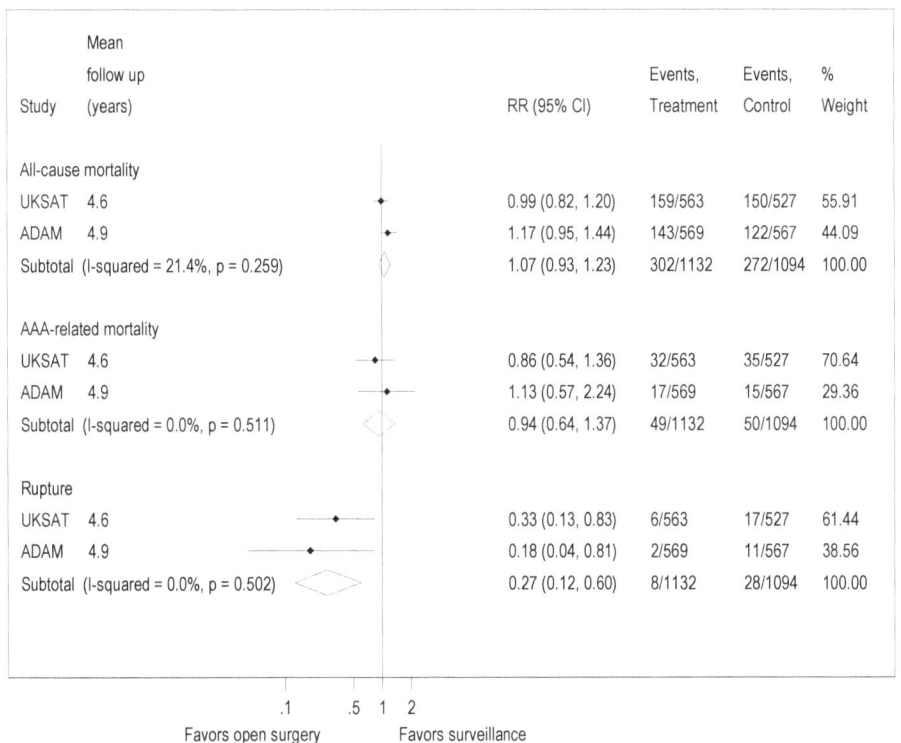

Study	Mean follow up (years)	RR (95% CI)	Events, Treatment	Events, Control	% Weight
All-cause mortality					
UKSAT	4.6	0.99 (0.82, 1.20)	159/563	150/527	55.91
ADAM	4.9	1.17 (0.95, 1.44)	143/569	122/567	44.09
Subtotal (I-squared = 21.4%, p = 0.259)		1.07 (0.93, 1.23)	302/1132	272/1094	100.00
AAA-related mortality					
UKSAT	4.6	0.86 (0.54, 1.36)	32/563	35/527	70.64
ADAM	4.9	1.13 (0.57, 2.24)	17/569	15/567	29.36
Subtotal (I-squared = 0.0%, p = 0.511)		0.94 (0.64, 1.37)	49/1132	50/1094	100.00
Rupture					
UKSAT	4.6	0.33 (0.13, 0.83)	6/563	17/527	61.44
ADAM	4.9	0.18 (0.04, 0.81)	2/569	11/567	38.56
Subtotal (I-squared = 0.0%, p = 0.502)		0.27 (0.12, 0.60)	8/1132	28/1094	100.00

.1   .5 1 2

Favors open surgery   Favors surveillance

Appendix K Figure 12. Pooled Analysis of Surgical Procedures to Repair AAA in Trials of Early Open Surgery or EVAR vs. Surveillance (KQ 5)

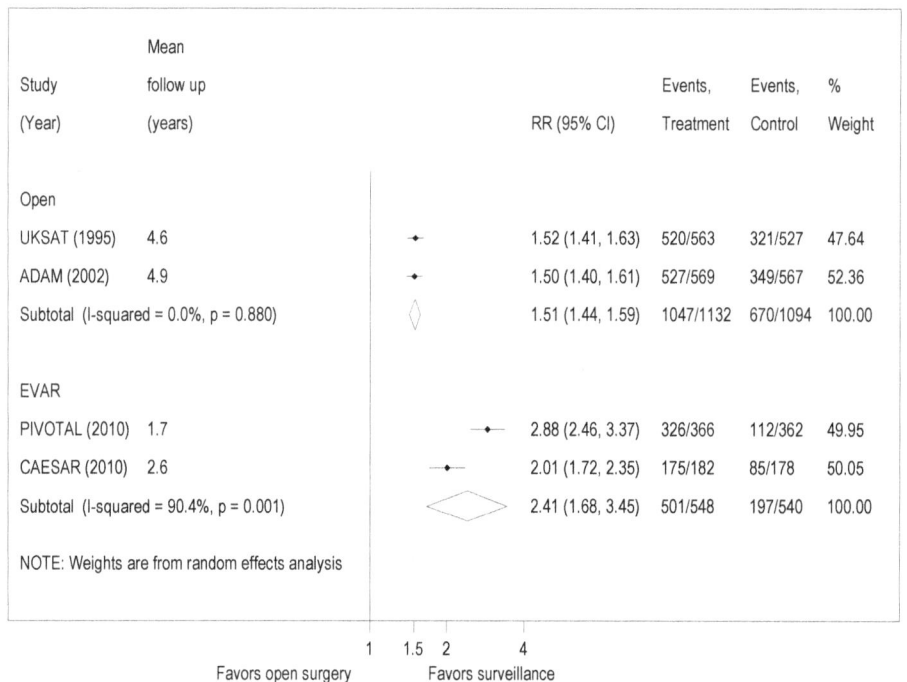

Study (Year)	Mean follow up (years)	RR (95% CI)	Events, Treatment	Events, Control	% Weight
Open					
UKSAT (1995)	4.6	1.52 (1.41, 1.63)	520/563	321/527	47.64
ADAM (2002)	4.9	1.50 (1.40, 1.61)	527/569	349/567	52.36
Subtotal (I-squared = 0.0%, p = 0.880)		1.51 (1.44, 1.59)	1047/1132	670/1094	100.00
EVAR					
PIVOTAL (2010)	1.7	2.88 (2.46, 3.37)	326/366	112/362	49.95
CAESAR (2010)	2.6	2.01 (1.72, 2.35)	175/182	85/178	50.05
Subtotal (I-squared = 90.4%, p = 0.001)		2.41 (1.68, 3.45)	501/548	197/540	100.00

NOTE: Weights are from random effects analysis

```
          1   1.5  2      4
Favors open surgery    Favors surveillance
```

Appendix K Figure 13. Pooled Analysis of All-Cause Mortality, AAA-Related Mortality, and Rupture in EVAR vs. Surveillance Trials (Fixed-Effects Model) (KQ 4)

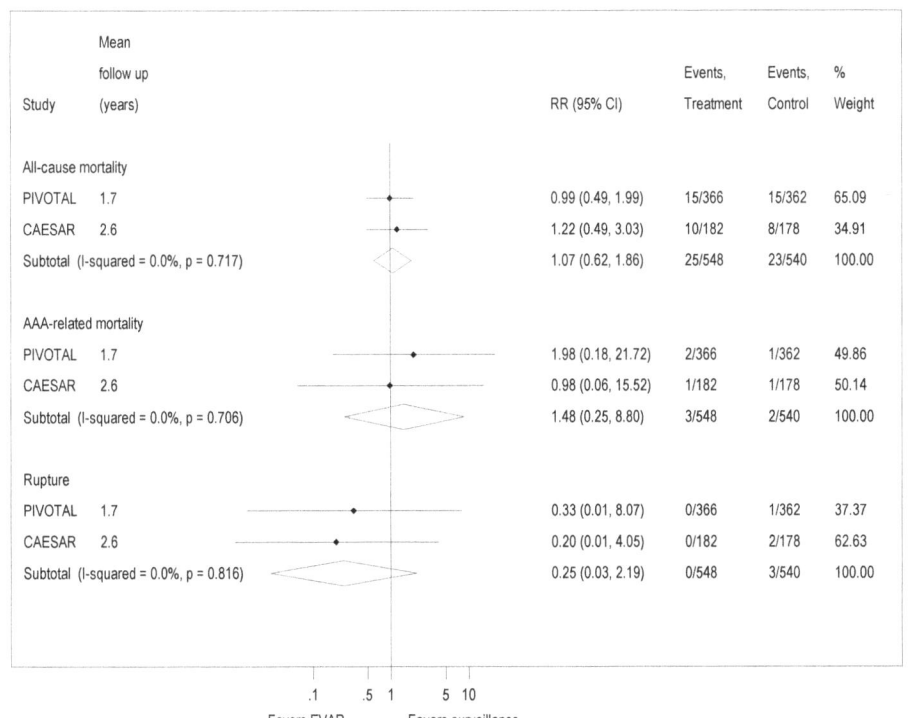

Study	Mean follow up (years)	RR (95% CI)	Events, Treatment	Events, Control	% Weight
All-cause mortality					
PIVOTAL	1.7	0.99 (0.49, 1.99)	15/366	15/362	65.09
CAESAR	2.6	1.22 (0.49, 3.03)	10/182	8/178	34.91
Subtotal (I-squared = 0.0%, p = 0.717)		1.07 (0.62, 1.86)	25/548	23/540	100.00
AAA-related mortality					
PIVOTAL	1.7	1.98 (0.18, 21.72)	2/366	1/362	49.86
CAESAR	2.6	0.98 (0.06, 15.52)	1/182	1/178	50.14
Subtotal (I-squared = 0.0%, p = 0.706)		1.48 (0.25, 8.80)	3/548	2/540	100.00
Rupture					
PIVOTAL	1.7	0.33 (0.01, 8.07)	0/366	1/362	37.37
CAESAR	2.6	0.20 (0.01, 4.05)	0/182	2/178	62.63
Subtotal (I-squared = 0.0%, p = 0.816)		0.25 (0.03, 2.19)	0/548	3/540	100.00

.1   .5   1   5   10
Favors EVAR   Favors surveillance

Appendix K Figure 14. Pooled Analysis of Surgical Procedures in Patients Receiving Pharmacotherapy vs. Placebo (KQ 5)

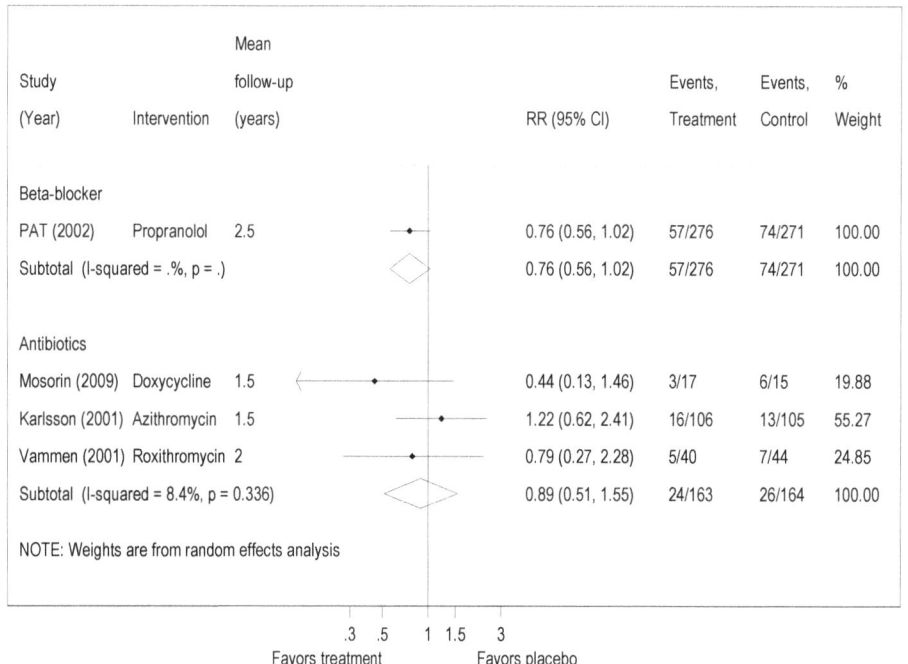

Study (Year)	Intervention	Mean follow-up (years)		RR (95% CI)	Events, Treatment	Events, Control	% Weight
Beta-blocker							
PAT (2002)	Propranolol	2.5		0.76 (0.56, 1.02)	57/276	74/271	100.00
Subtotal (I-squared = .%, p = .)				0.76 (0.56, 1.02)	57/276	74/271	100.00
Antibiotics							
Mosorin (2009)	Doxycycline	1.5		0.44 (0.13, 1.46)	3/17	6/15	19.88
Karlsson (2001)	Azithromycin	1.5		1.22 (0.62, 2.41)	16/106	13/105	55.27
Vammen (2001)	Roxithromycin	2		0.79 (0.27, 2.28)	5/40	7/44	24.85
Subtotal (I-squared = 8.4%, p = 0.336)				0.89 (0.51, 1.55)	24/163	26/164	100.00

NOTE: Weights are from random effects analysis

.3   .5   1   1.5   3
Favors treatment   Favors placebo

Appendix K Figure 15. Pooled Analysis of All-Cause Mortality in Trials of Antibiotics vs. Placebo (Fixed-Effects Model) (KQ 4)

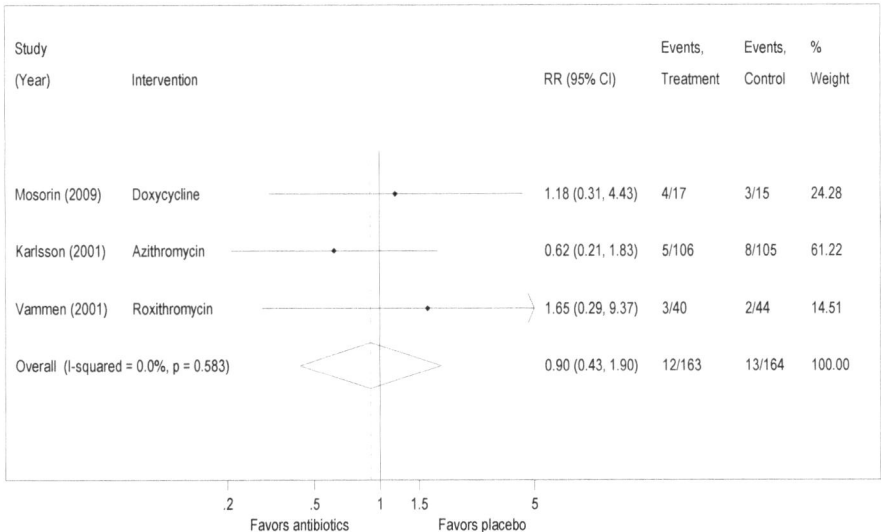

Study (Year)	Intervention	RR (95% CI)	Events, Treatment	Events, Control	% Weight
Mosorin (2009)	Doxycycline	1.18 (0.31, 4.43)	4/17	3/15	24.28
Karlsson (2001)	Azithromycin	0.62 (0.21, 1.83)	5/106	8/105	61.22
Vammen (2001)	Roxithromycin	1.65 (0.29, 9.37)	3/40	2/44	14.51
Overall (I-squared = 0.0%, p = 0.583)		0.90 (0.43, 1.90)	12/163	13/164	100.00

.2   .5   1   1.5   5

Favors antibiotics   Favors placebo

www.ingramcontent.com/pod-product-compliance
Lightning Source LLC
Chambersburg PA
CBHW081725170526

45167CB00009B/3706